With Love

Sheron

Oliver Howard

THE FAT HANDLE

From lo-carb to NO-carb

Typeset in Linotype Optima®
Printed by createspace.com

Published by Oliver Howard MMXIV
v.1.0.2
with minor corrections

ISBN 978-0-9930155-3-3

CONTENTS

INTRODUCTION

This is a very simple book:

- I have been overweight for 20 years and obese for 10.

- I have tried everything they say we should do to lose weight.

- Nothing worked; in the end it only made me fatter.

- Then I tried an idea of my own.

- It worked.

- Now I am telling you about it.

That's it, really. I claim no specialist knowledge and simply know what I know from books I have read (many of which are listed in the appendix) and especially from things I have done myself. It often feels like a lot of weight advice comes from people who have been skinny all their lives and have no real idea what it's like to struggle with overweight and obesity.

But if I say something in this book you don't believe, then go and check it out for yourself. Don't just say "I don't believe it." Be curious, see if there are others who agree with me. It'll be the easiest thing in the world to find people who disagree, but scratch a little deeper and you'll find plenty others who say what I am saying.

Or try it out for yourself. Remember, the Earth isn't flat, or at the centre of the Universe, as people used to be told very firmly to believe. Look around you and draw your own conclusions.

One of the things I have come to realise is how different we all are. Many of the ways I have tried to lose weight work for others but not for me. So what I am telling you here may not work for you. There's no one-size-fits-all.

But if you are like me and have tried everything else short of surgery, you'll want to try this. Because it might work, and if it does, you're on your way to a lighter, healthier life. For good. No more yo-yoing, no more embarrassment, no more nightly heartburn, no more messing around with diets that don't work.

You'll have found the handle that controls your weight. I call it the fat handle.

Oliver Howard

1. How we get fat

We are told all the time that gaining or losing weight is a simple game of numbers. Numbers of calories. If you eat more calories than you use then you gain weight, and if you eat fewer calories than you use then you lose weight.

I wish. And I bet that so do you.

No doubt this is a very fine theory, but it ignores the complexity of our metabolism and how it messes up that simple logic. It may work for weight *gain*, but weight loss is not simply weight gain in reverse as seems to be the conventional thinking.

Besides, this book is not so much about how to keep from getting fat but more about what to do once you are, and the experience of countless people trying desperately to lose weight—and keep it off— shows that it's not that simple. If it were, then dieting would not be such a huge industry and obesity would not be the health problem it is.

Don't know about you, but I have always been able to lose 10 pounds or so on a low calorie diet. But absolutely no more. When I've lost those 10 pounds, my body starts reacting to getting fewer calories than it needs, and by whatever metabolic trickery I then can't lose any more weight no matter how much I starve myself.

And of course I can only keep that up for so long. Then when I go back to eating normally, I gradually gain not 10 pounds but 12. It is as if my body got such a shock from starving that it now wants to put even more aside for next time.

I should mention here that "eating normally" for me doesn't mean gorging on huge portions or stuffing myself with junk food. I'm the cook in the family and I make most things from scratch. No processed meals here but proper food made mostly from fresh ingredients, preferably organic and many self-grown, and in sensible amounts. I have had precisely two fast food meals in the last ten years and I don't drink things full of sugar. I don't even use the stuff in my tea.

I say this, not to be holier-than-thou but to point out that the reasons we get fat aren't as simple as many weight gurus would have us believe.

Then there's the other argument: eating fat makes you fat. Yeah, right, like drinking water makes you all runny? There's more to our metabolism than this simple "you are what you eat" mantra. But we believe it, in our droves, and we buy tons of low fat food as a result. Food with less fat, but the problem is that it has more of something else, and that something else is positively deadly: SUGAR.

Which brings me to why we get fat.

Everything we eat ends up in our stomach where it is digested. This is where it gets interesting, because what digestion does is break down the nutrients in the food so they can be absorbed into the bloodstream. There are three main groups of nutrients: carbohydrates, fat and protein.

I won't be dealing with the details of fat and protein here because they play little role in the fat that gets stored away in our fat cells. It is now accepted that *eating fat does not make us fat*, and Dr. Ancel Keys' "Seven Countries" study which started that wild goose chase 50 years ago is now widely discredited as bad science. For details, please see the books referred to in the appendix.

It's the carbohydrates that are key to weight gain and loss, and this is how it works. There are many different kinds of carbs, but our digestion breaks them all down into exactly the same stuff: glucose. Which is sugar to you and me, and that goes straight into the blood.

Let me say that again, because it is the most important single piece of information in this book and the key to everything else, so you really must get your head around it: ALL carbohydrates we eat end up in the blood as glucose, or blood sugar.

It doesn't matter if they come from supposedly healthy things or from the worst junk food, or even pure, refined sugar. OK, there is one exception, which is fibre, because it is not digested but passes through us unchanged, but even the best full grain products have plenty of digestible carbohydrate beside the fibre. That is all turned into sugar by our digestion.

So far that's not a problem. Glucose is a super efficient way to get energy to where our body needs it. The trouble starts when we eat more carbohydrates than we need just at that moment. Then our blood sugar level starts to rise, and that would damage our body if nothing was done about it because too much sugar is harmful to cells.

Even that is not a problem provided you are not diabetic. For most people it just means that their pancreas starts to produce a hormone called insulin, and that hormone starts to remove the excess sugar from the blood.

And guess how. It turns it into fat which it stuffs into the fat cells in our bodies. Well, first it stores excess glucose as *glycogen* in the liver and muscles, but when those stores are full, the rest is stored as fat. So every time you eat more carbohydrates than your body immediately needs for energy, you get a little fatter.

But even that is fine. In fact, it is our survival mechanism for lean times, because when you *don't* get enough carbohydrates, then the process runs in reverse. The fat stored in your fat cells turns into glucose which enters the bloodstream and is used for energy. Magic.

Only problem is that this reverse process won't get going as long as there is too much insulin in the blood, because the role of insulin is to *store* fat, so it prevents its release. And, of course, there is insulin in the blood as long as there more glucose there than is immediately needed.

To make matters worse, as we get fatter, a phenomenon called insulin resistance sets in (the main mechanism in type 2 diabetes). This makes insulin levels go even higher, blocking the release of fat for energy at even lower levels of blood glucose.

So here we are: we store fat as a way to store energy for later use, but that fat is never released and used for energy as long as insulin levels remain too high. Net result: the fat stays in the cells and we keep piling on the pounds, little by little.

2. How we lose the fat

I did not invent or discover the process I describe in chapter 1. I read about it in a lot of other books, some of which are listed in the appendix. I didn't invent ways to reverse that process, either. Others did, and you can read about them in those books, too.

What I DID find out, however, is that those ways don't work for me, and thereby hangs a tale which is at least as important as anything to do with my weight, so please bear with me.

Most of my life I have suffered from respiratory infections. Everything from sore throats to bronchitis and pneumonia, and I had them 3, 4 or 5 times a year.

But then I also did something that perhaps I shouldn't have done. I drank a lot of milk. People told me that wasn't good for me, so in 2001 I stopped drinking milk, just to see if that would make a difference. Voila! My throat infections stopped and I haven't had one since.

That was great, of course, but then the following year I got bronchitis three times and in between those I had pneumonia twice. It was as if infections, no longer taking hold in my throat, had free access further down my airways.

The first pneumonia, in the spring, was double sided but bacterial, so it responded to antibiotics but still took months to get over. In the autumn I got pneumonia again, and this time it was viral which means antibiotics didn't work. I was already weakened from two attacks of bronchitis within a short space of time plus the previous pneumonia, so if this viral pneumonia had been double sided, I might not have survived. I was 52 years old.

Luckily my last pneumonia was single sided and I recovered, only to finish off the year with a third bout of bronchitis. All that left me deeply shaken, both physically and mentally. I had to do something or I feared I wouldn't get to 60.

Then my wife told me about a book she had read, and suggested I read it. It was called *Life Without Bread*, and I don't think I exaggerate if I say that book saved my life.

I'm not going to try to tell you everything that's in it but I strongly recommend you read it yourself. Suffice to say that it deals in great detail with the health effects of eating too many carbohydrates. On the strength of that and a few other books, I cut, not milk this time, but nearly all the rest of the carbohydrates I was eating: bread, potatoes, pasta and rice.

In other words I started eating low-carb, as was becoming fashionable at the time.

For me, that was like throwing a switch. My immune system kicked into action, and in the 12 years since then I have had bronchitis once, but not very seriously. In the 20 or 30 years before that I had one respiratory infection or another four times a year on average, so the difference is there for anyone to see.

That was wonderful, of course, so the fact that I didn't lose weight eating low-carb, like all the celebrities, didn't bother me too much at the time.

Fast forward 12 years. Still healthy, but also still overweight. Nay, obese, with a BMI pushing 35. My blood pressure, cholesterol and other vital statistics were fine, but I knew my obesity meant I was at increased risk of heart problems and diabetes, and maybe even some types of cancer. Types of cancer people around me were dying from.

It was also hard to buy decent clothes, and more and more aspects of life were getting to be a drag. On top of that there's the social stigma. Fat people are increasingly looked down on as losers and scroungers on society. They are seen as being out of control, and we hear more and more about the costs, especially to a health system buckling under the weight of an obesity epidemic.

For all those reasons, and many more, I was getting desperate to find a way to fight the flab that would work for me. I had read the books listed in the appendix and was convinced that there was a link between eating too much carbohydrate and obesity, but I had cut the carbs and nothing had happened to my weight.

So I started thinking. Since a lot of people lose weight on low-carb diets, why wasn't it working for me? Assuming it's true that we can't take fat out of storage while there is too much insulin in the blood, then an obvious question is: *how much is too much?*

Could it be that the insulin level at which the fat process can run in reverse is different for different people? Why not? So many other things are different for different people, so why should this be the same for everybody? The more I thought about it, the more it made sense.

Not only that, but the simpler it seemed to check if it was true. I just had to reduce carbs *even more* than I already had and watch what would happen.

So I decided to go from *lo-carb* to *no-carb*, or as near as I could get. Even the greenest of greens have small amounts of carbohydrates in them, but when I did my sums it looked like I could bring my carb intake below 10 grams a day.

That's half of what even the most restrictive low-carb diets prescribe, and I couldn't get lower while eating normal, healthy and tasty food. I didn't want to start eating in a way that was either going to affect my health or that I hated so much that I couldn't keep it up. I had tried that before and didn't want to go there again.

To keep it simple to begin with, I decided to eat only eggs, fish, meat and low carb vegetables and drink nothing but water, tea and coffee. I knew I could keep that up for a while to see what happened.

And this is what happened to my BMI over the next two weeks:

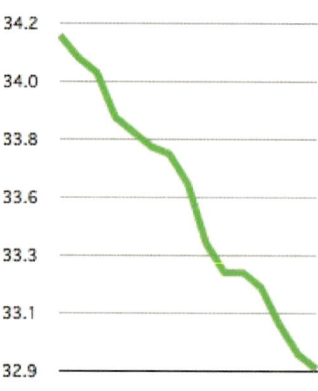

First two weeks' weight loss in BMI

Expressed as weight this is 10 pounds, which is an impressive enough weight loss for two weeks, but what was just as eye-popping was the sheer slope of the curve. This was weight loss as I had never seen it before, and whenever it threatened to level out I had a pretty good idea why, which meant I could quickly do something about it.

To me that felt like finding a handle that controlled my weight, for the first time ever. What's more, it was fitting in with health professionals beginning to talk about *metabolic types* (see chapter 4).

My weight kept plummeting at the same rate for the next two weeks, by which time I had lost 20 pounds. Then I hit a few bumps, but it was mainly because I had started relaxing a bit, so I just had to learn to control that.

By then I had started fitting clothes I had not worn for years, the nighttime heartburn had stopped and I was beginning to like what I saw in the mirror, so the motivation to continue was sky-high. Was it hard to get back on the straight and narrow? You bet it wasn't!

You can see from the next curve that the first four weeks were the easiest. Then there were some ups and downs the next couple of months, often because I started adding a few things back into what I ate or drank. While it wasn't hard to eat the way I did, I wanted to eat as "normally" and varied as possible, and it didn't take much to upset the balance.

I know the weight gurus tell us only to look at our weight once a week, but to me the daily records are an important tool in spotting trouble and dealing with it and that way keep the momentum going.

And you know what? I didn't think I owed a thing, least of all respect, to people whose advice had done me no good for 20 years or more. For me this daily table is an essential tool that helps me stay focused.

I'm using a simple spreadsheet I made myself, but there are plenty of fancy apps out there that will do it for you and work out your BMI at the same time.

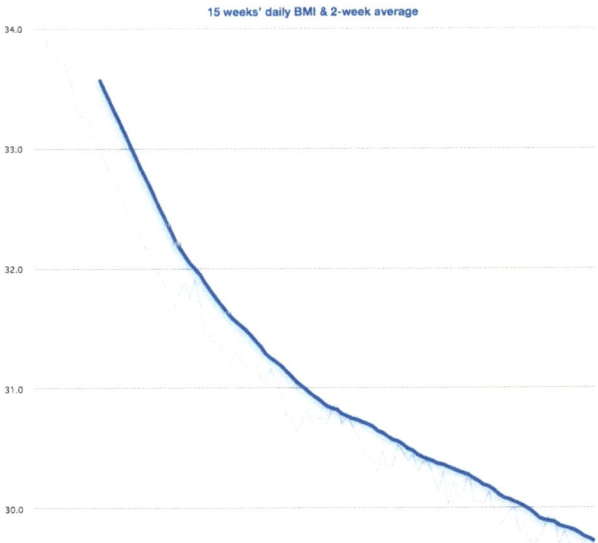

The thin line is my daily BMI curve, the thick line is the 14-day average which removes the bumps. That's what the curve would have looked like if I had only checked my weight every two weeks, except that then I would have missed early signs of trouble and not been able to make timely corrections.

Just to make sure that I wasn't doing myself any harm, I had a thorough health check and a good discussion of the details of my no-carb regime with my doctor after the first four weeks. Everything was fine, blood pressure and blood tests never better, and I was cleared to continue as I had begun.

I strongly recommend that you do the same, especially if your weight loss is significant, and if you have health issues other than your weight you simply must do it.

While no-carb eating deprives you of absolutely nothing essential for a healthy life, as is documented in the literature listed in the appendix, it is important to remember that we are all different, and your body may react differently to losing weight at this rate.

See your doctor after the first few weeks and make sure you're not doing yourself an injury.

Slimming pills

Why go through all this, you might ask. Why not just pop a few pills as plenty of adverts tell you to do? Here's why.

Slimming pills—at least those that have any effect at all—work by blocking the digestion of some of the carbohydrates or fats in your food. In other words, even if you eat more of it than you need, it doesn't all end up in your bloodstream.

Great. As long as it lasts. I've done it, and I did lose weight, but as soon as I stopped taking the pills, it all came back and then some. Sounds familiar?

The reason is that I did not change my eating habits, and that is ultimately what I have to do if I am to stay at a lower weight. The pills didn't need me to change what I ate, in fact that was one of their selling points, so why should I?

No-carb eating, on the other hand, got me used to eating differently, simply by being aware of what I put into my body. Of course I won't have to eat no-carb for the rest of my life, because I don't want to keep losing weight forever, but when I go from weight loss to weight maintenance, it is a simple matter of adding some selected carbs back into my diet.

Using the fat handle.

I also find the idea of eating things and then putting chemicals into my body to make those things pass straight through me not only bizarre but also worrying. Do I know everything those chemicals do to me? Of course I don't. I did find out some of the more obvious side effects though, such as what fat blocking pills did to my digestion. Dealing with the resulting sticky, oily, orange mess is not something I recommend, but to me it's just as important that losing weight this way doesn't work in the long run.

No-carb works because you get a grip on what you eat, and in the next chapter we'll look at how to use that for long term weight management.

Conventional slimming

Another alternative to eating no-carb is conventional slimming with its combination of a low calorie diet and exercise. Not a word against exercise, it's good for us for all sorts of reasons, and we should do as much of it as we can fit into our busy lives.

Slimming is just not one of those reasons as found in recent studies which show that exercise has very little effect on weight loss. First of all it takes an awful lot of exercise to burn a decent amount of calories (a full hour's energetic jogging will burn fewer than 500 calories), and a lot of that calorie burn is offset by eating more after exercise because appetite increases with activity.

Note that this does NOT mean you might as well be a couch potato. All it means is that exercise is just not a viable way to lose weight.

The following curves shows what happened to me when I tried to lose weight through exercise and traditional dieting over a period of more than a year about ten years ago, compared to what no-carb eating did in four months just recently:

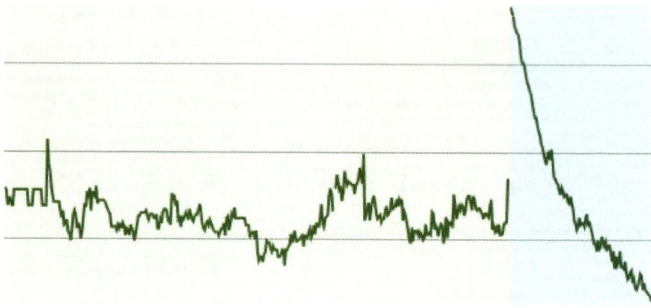

Green background: conventional slimming, blue background: no-carb eating

The curve to the right shows some jitters as my weight drops off, but it still maintains a clear downward direction. That was never the case with conventional slimming, which shows the ups and downs so familiar to anyone who has tried to shed the pounds over any length of time.

3. How we keep off the fat

This book is mainly about understanding why we get fat and then giving you a tool to lose that fat, but clearly a diet that loses you several pounds a week is not something you want to keep up forever.

So once you've reached the weight, or BMI, you want to be at, the question is how do you stop the weight loss and stay there?

The answer is simple: start adding back into your diet some of the things you removed in order to lose weight and then keep an eye on what happens. If your weight keeps going down, you should add more, and if it starts going up again you need to cut some of the things you just added. What could be simpler and healthier?

That mechanism is what I call my *fat handle*. You now have a grip on your weight so IT no longer controls YOU but the other way around.

So what should you add? Entirely up to you. If it's bread or pasta or chocolate or beer doesn't really matter from a weight point of view. You'll want to consider health issues other than just weight, of course, but now that you know that carbohydrates, and to some extent alcohol, are the key to your weight, you can find the variety and amounts of food that suit you and keep your weight where you want it.

For me, that's a mix of things. A croissant may creep back into Sunday breakfasts, and rice or potatoes will occasionally appear on the dinner plate again. Definitely a glass of wine and a drink now and then. But the point is that we can all make our own decisions.

What you absolutely don't want to do is go back to your old eating habits. If you do that, you'll have done all this for nothing, and the pounds will just pile back on. Keep an eye on those scales and do something about it as soon as your weight starts changing.

If it goes up, and you're anything like me, you'll know immediately what you have done to make that happen, and my advice is to do something just as immediately to correct it.

If it goes down, add more of your favourite carbs. You don't want to end up anorexic, which is a real danger for people who focus too much on their weight. Decide on the weight that's right for you and stay close to that.

With the fat handle, you are in control of where you want to be on the scales. It's like the accelerator in a car: if you start going faster than you want, you don't wait until you're out of control before you back off a little. You do it immediately.

Use your fat handle like the accelerator in your car to keep your weight under control.

As your new eating habits stabilise your weight, you can relax your weighing regime and only check it once a week as they tell us to do, and later even once a month. Daily fluctuations can present a confusing picture for weight maintenance, but if your long term weight starts changing, up or down, you now have the tool you need to bring it back where you want it.

Your own, personal fat handle.

4. The devil in the detail

BMI - OLD AND NEW

BMI stands for Body Mass Index and is a way to express normal weight, underweight and overweight independently of a person's height.

The index is calculated by dividing the body weight in kilograms by the square of the height in metres:

BMI = KG / M²

E.g. $65 / 1.75^2 = 21.2$

In imperial measures it gets a little more messy but works the same way:

BMI = (LB / IN²) x 703

E.g. $(145 / 69^2) \times 703 = 21.4$

You'll be glad to know that there are plenty of BMI calculators, both online and as apps for pads and phones, so you don't have to do the maths yourself. Some of them can even keep records and make pretty graphs.

BMIs from 18.5 to 25 are considered normal, while less than 18.5 is underweight, more than 25 is overweight and more than 30 is obese. Outside those values there are ranges for both severe underweight and severe obesity.

BMIs in this book are based on this calculation because it's been around for a long time and people know it, but there is a problem with it for people who don't fit into a fairly narrow range of heights. It doesn't work for children or short adults, and tall people need to be comparatively thinner for the same BMI.

This is because the index varies with the *square* of the height, while a body would grow by the *cube* of the height, were it to maintain the same proportions. But our bodies aren't simple geometrical shapes and they don't just change proportionally in all directions, so varying the BMI with the cube of the height wouldn't work either.

Professor L. N. Trefethen, head of the University of Oxford's numerical analysis group, said in a letter published in the Economist in January 2013 that the BMI:

> ...was invented in the 1840s, before calculators, when a formula had to be very simple to be usable. As a consequence of this ill-founded definition, millions of short people think they are thinner than they are, and millions of tall people think they are fatter.

Indeed, the inventor of the BMI (then called the Quetelet Index), Belgian mathematician and sociologist Adolphe Quetelet, did discuss this issue in his *Treatise on Man and the Development of his Faculties* published in 1842, but he still chose to base his index on the simple square of the height. Possibly because the more complex math needed for a better fit to real human bodies was not easily performed by many people back then, and he wanted his index to become widely used.

However, in an age of calculators, computers and smart gadgets, Professor Trefethen saw no need to keep things simple at the cost of accuracy. He therefore proposed a new BMI calculation which takes into account differences in the proportions of people of various heights:

New BMI = (KG x 1.3) / M$^{2.5}$

E.g. $(65 \times 1.3) / 1.75^{2.5} = 20.9$

or, in pounds and inches:

New BMI = (LB / IN$^{2.5}$) x 5734

E.g. $(145 / 69^{2.5}) \times 5734 = 20.9$

By this calculation, someone 15 cm or 6 inches shorter than average would gain 0.6 points on a BMI of 21 and someone 15 cm taller than average would lose 1.2 points.

Expressed in weight, the shorter person should be 1.5 kilos or just over 3 pounds lighter, and the taller person 4.5 kilos or 10 pounds heavier, for a BMI of 21.

The following web link takes you to an online calculator which works out both old and new BMIs for metric as well as imperial measurements:

http://people.maths.ox.ac.uk/trefethen/bmi_calc.html

Even with this complexity, as the calculator warns in its footnote:

...the new BMI, like the old BMI, is just a single number, and no single number can capture the complexity of our bodies and associated health issues.

Still, the BMI, old or new, is useful for comparisons and as an aiming point. You just have to decide for yourself where you want to be on the "normal" scale of 18.5 to 25.

Especially with the old index, a tall person is likely to be most comfortable at the higher end of the scale and a smaller person towards the lower end.

Carbs, kidney stones and heartburn

Unfortunately the advice on kidney stones and diet is unclear. Some say that a diet high in protein can increase kidney stone problems and others say that it makes no difference.

What no-one says is that a diet low in carbohydrates in itself has any effect one way or the other on kidney stones, but when you eat fewer carbs, you naturally increase the proportion of protein in your food, which leads us back to the first, unresolved, question.

However, it's probably fair to say that if you do have kidney stone problems, especially if they are significant, you should talk to your doctor before embarking on a no-carb, and therefore high-protein, diet.

My personal experience is that a slight kidney stone problem has completely disappeared after I started my no-carb diet, most likely not as a direct result but as an indirect consequence. With my earlier diet, I had frequent heartburn, especially at night, and periodically used antacids. That heartburn has completely disappeared with my new no-carb food, and I therefore don't need the antacids any more.

I know that correlation does not prove causation, but on the other hand I see no other reason why my kidney stone problem should have gone away precisely at the same time I started no-carb eating and stopped using antacids. Unless it is the no-carb diet that does it, and no-one is claiming that.

Apparently the problem is especially with antacids containing calcium, so beware of those if you have difficulties with kidney stones.

Glucose, insulin and ketones

All the cells in our body need energy to function, and most of them get that energy from glucose in the blood, so there's nothing bad about blood glucose as such. The trouble comes, as mentioned earlier, when glucose levels are frequently so high that the excess gets stored away as fat, and when that process is not allowed to run "in reverse," allowing that fat to be used as fuel later on.

It is the insulin hormone that removes excess glucose from the blood and stores it as fat, and it's insulin that prevents the fat from being taken out of storage again, so long as the insulin level is being kept high by high levels of glucose and/or by insulin resistance.

It is easy to see that this evil circle can be broken by eating less carbohydrate, but *how much less* is not so clear. Many books will tell you that 20 to 50 grams a day will make you lose weight, and that is true for many people. Good for them.

I just wasn't one of them, and if you have come this far, then chances are that you aren't either. So I drew the logical conclusion that 20 or 50 grams was still too much for me and decided to see what happened if I reduced it even more.

That is the ONLY part of this book I have invented myself, but even if that is unscientific and hearsay and not a proof and whatever else people will call it in order to rubbish it, I believe my results speak for themselves.

However, that still leaves a question about how a body functions when it is denied the very fuel it runs on, so I'll explain that briefly but refer you to the literature in the appendix for full details.

There are two ways: the body can make the glucose it needs for energy from its own stores of glycogen, or when they are depleted from fatty acids ("fat" to you and me). This process is called *gluconeogenesis,* and it is what I call "burning the fat."

The other way is called *ketosis,* and before anyone gets into a flap about that, let me explain that ketosis is *not* the same as *ketoacidosis.* The latter is a serious condition associated with uncontrolled diabetes, and all it has in common with ketosis are elevated levels of *ketones* in the blood. However, ketone levels associated with ketoacidosis are 5 to 10 times higher than for ketosis, in fact so high that the blood becomes acidic.

Ketosis, on the other hand, is a natural and healthy condition in which the body in a controlled way turns fatty acids into ketones instead of glucose, and those ketones are then used for fuel. It takes a few days for cells, especially brain cells, to adjust to using ketones for energy instead of glucose, but after that the body functions equally well on ketones.

So will you be in ketosis on a no-carb diet or will you live on gluconeogenesis? Well, that appears to depend on how your body works —again, we're not all the same. For instance, I do not go into ketosis, no matter how little carbohydrate I eat. My ketone levels are normal, i.e. 0.2-0.3 mmol/L, about a tenth of what they would be if I were in ketosis.

And my glucose levels are also normal: somewhere between 4.5 and 5.3 mmol/L no matter what time of day or night, or if it's before or after a meal. I simply don't have the "sugar highs" and "lows" we get when eating carbohydrates, but just the right level of glucose in my blood that I need at any one time.

The only place this glucose can come from is gluconeogenesis, in other words my body is making its own glucose from stores of fatty acids. The reason this process works is that the level of insulin is low enough to allow it to take place.

That's how I lose weight, but others will do that via ketosis. Either way, it doesn't matter: you are using your stored fat for energy, and you don't have to worry about or monitor it. I just did that because this was new and interesting and I wanted to understand it and be able to explain to others what was going on.

However, for those who do want to keep an eye their glucose, and possibly ketone, levels, I have included in the appendix a link to a monitoring system that will do both.

To sum up: your body will get the energy it needs from its own energy stores, and the reason that works is that the insulin is kept low enough for the fat to be taken out of storage as nature intended.

That's the process explained in layman's terms, but check out the books in the appendix for more highbrow detail.

Lifestyle

This heading is not a way to sneak in a lecture on the virtues of exercise and clean living or throw accusations at you about your level of activity. By all means get all the exercise you can, I do and it's good for a lot of reasons, but this book is about something else.

No, what I mean by lifestyle is that I know that I don't live my life like most people, and of course that has an impact on what I find it easy to eat while others may find it more difficult.

For one thing I usually have time in the morning to sit and enjoy my breakfast and drink a pot of tea while I read a book or catch up with the news. I also normally have time for a decent lunch break and I'm often near my own kitchen and can cook things fresh, even in the middle of the day.

Lucky me, but then I do work late into the evenings when the rest of the world has gone quiet. My point is that the fact that your day is different to mine doesn't mean you can't eat no-carb. You'll just have to figure out a way that works for you.

Getting a no-carb lunch may be the biggest challenge for many people with a busy life, so I have included in the picture cookbook a number of simple salads which you can prepare in the morning, or the night before, and refrigerate until lunchtime. If you can't keep them cool that long, make sure you're using things that won't go off (more on that in chapter 6). Take your inspiration from these dishes and create more of your own, using your favourite low-carb ingredients chosen from the lists in chapter 5.

Or choose among the meat, fish, egg and vegetable items where you normally get your lunch. Leave the bread, beans, rice, pizza and pasta behind, and especially the sweets and "energy" bars and drinks and all the other junk food.

If you can't get anything but a sandwich, get two or three, eat the filling and treat the bread as wrapping. I know that would be expensive and wasteful, but at least it's good for you.

Leaving your cooking to others comes with risks though, because you have no control over what they put in it, especially in terms of sweeteners and additives, some of which may push up insulin levels and therefore work against weight loss. Eating home cooked food made from quality ingredients is the only way to know for sure what you are putting into your body.

Metabolic types

Many health professionals are now beginning to talk about something they call *metabolic types*, meaning that we don't all need the same food any more than all cars can run on the same fuel. In fact, that is a useful analogy because the food we eat is exactly that: the fuel that our body runs on.

One such doctor describes how a large part of his patients did not respond, or responded negatively, to his dietary advice. At first he thought it was because those patients didn't follow his counsel (the standard, arrogant derision of patients as naughty children), but when he examined his own preconceptions, he found that in fact most of them did. Something else was going on.

He eventually came to the conclusion that what was wrong was the one-size-fits-all advice he was giving them, so he instead started analysing his his patients' metabolic types and basing his health and weight advice on the results.

It turns out that some people live best on high-carbohydrate food which they metabolise effectively into energy, while they have difficulty metabolising protein and fat which therefore cause them problems. People at the other end of the scale live best on protein and fat, and carbohydrates cause them major health and weight problems. In the middle is a group that needs a mix of the two.

Of course, there aren't just three distinct groups but a wide spectrum with two extremes and endless variation between these poles. But what this approach is beginning to recognise is *that we are not all the same,* which is precisely the idea that made me cut the carbohydrates to near-zero because maybe, just maybe, I was more sensitive to insulin than most other people.

As I have said before in this book, no-carb eating is not for everyone. It's for that group of the population who don't tolerate carbs well, but then, if you weren't in that group, you'd be unlikely to read this. Because eating carbohydrates is what everybody has been telling you to do, and look where that got you. You need to start eating the food that your body runs best on.

Look at like this: If you had a car and didn't know or care if it was petrol or diesel, would you CONTINUE to fill it with diesel if, time and time again, it had conked out when you did?

Salt

We are constantly told to cut down on salt because it's bad for us. The reason is that we're expected to eat lots of processed food which is stuffed full of it. Nearly all processed food, from bread and cheese to burgers and pies, has a high salt content, so no wonder it's a job keeping down the amount of salt you eat if this is what you mostly live on.

What we rarely hear is that without salt, we would die. And when you prepare your own no-carb food from fresh ingredients, as I do, it only contains the salt that you add to it yourself. There is no salt in things like broccoli, cauliflower, chicken, beef or salmon. There is some in ham, but nothing like in most bread.

So how much salt should you add to your no-carb food? Salt, chemically known as sodium chloride, consists of 40% sodium and 60% chlorine by weight. The minimum amount of sodium to sustain life is 500 mg per day, so this translates to 1.3 g of salt. However, the *recommended* daily intake for healthy adults is 1500 mg of sodium, or close to 4 grams of salt, to replace the amount lost through sweat and urine.

The maximum recommended daily dose of sodium is 2300 mg (6 g salt), so this is something you want to measure out quite carefully.

6 g of salt is just under a teaspoonful, or 5 c.c. but I have found that an easier and far more practical way to measure salt is in *pinches*. Not the metaphoric pinch of salt with which we should take many things, but literally the amount of salt I can pinch between my thumb, index and middle fingers. No matter if this is fine table salt or coarse sea salt crystals, experiments show that what I pick up in a three-finger pinch is very close to one gram.

So the smallest amount of salt I should add per day to my (otherwise salt free) food is a-pinch-and-a-bit, but the recommended amount is four pinches, and I should not exceed six pinches.

In reality one pinch per meal, or three a day, turns out to be what I like. Any more than that I find my food too salty, any less too bland. If you look carefully at some of the pictures in chapter 6, you can spot the coarse crystals of my favourite sea salt.

Adding the salt I like feels positively rebellious, and liberating, after everything we have been told about avoiding it, but it makes sense when you think about it.

What to drink and not to drink

When I cut out the carbs, I also cut out the alcohol. All alcohol: wine, beer, strong spirits, the lot. And every time I have tried to add small amounts back in, it upsets my weight loss enough for me to quit again. That's one of the reasons I like to keep daily records.

I couldn't understand why this happened, because there aren't any carbohydrates in neat alcohol, so except for beer and sweet wine, it shouldn't be a problem. But when I looked hard enough, I found evidence that alcohol is linked to increased insulin secretion. That would explain why someone like me, who clearly has to have very low insulin levels for the fat burning process to work, can't mix alcohol with weight loss.

So I'm on the wagon? Yes, but even if I like a drink as much as the next fellow, it's a small sacrifice. At the same time it's good for my body in all sorts of other ways, not just weight. And it's not forever; when I get to the weight I want to maintain, alcohol is one of the things I am going to allow back into my diet.

I drink mostly water while I eat no-carb, and lots of it. Up to a litre with every meal—breakfast, lunch and dinner—plus smaller amounts in between. Tea and coffee count as water, just don't lace it with sweeteners or lashings of milk. If you take your coffee white, use real cream.

But then that's not very different from what I did before I went no-carb. I've had my big pot of tea in the morning for more than 20 years, and a jug of ice water with lunch for more than 10, ever since I gave up milk. It's mostly the wine with dinner and the occasional drink afterwards I've given up.

Of course, I have no sweetened drinks at all. Although they look fairly innocent in the carbohydrate tables in chapter 5, the danger with liquids is that we consume a lot more of them than we do solids. So even if a Coke, with around 10 g of carbs per 100 ml, looks benign compared to white bread with around 45 g, a single can still contains as many carbs as five slices of toast (35 g).

Similarly for milk. Only 5 g carbs per 100 ml - but beware. Drink a litre and you might as well spoon down 50 grams of refined sugar, and who would think of doing such a thing?

5. Carbohydrate tables

The following tables list the digestible (net) carbohydrate contents for over 500 common foodstuffs. Non-digestible carbs (fibres) are not counted as they are not digested and therefore do not affect blood sugar or insulin levels.

The numbers in the tables are grams of carbohydrate per 100 grams of the food, or per 100 ml for liquids. In other words, they are percentages.

The tables are colour coded as follows:

Green	Less than 5% carbohydrates
Yellow	5% or more but less than 10%
Orange	10% or more but less than 20%
Red	20% or more
Purple	Alcohol

There are two tables, each with the same information, but arranged differently.

The first table is sorted into groups of food—dairy, fruit, meat, vegetables and so on—then alphabetically within each group to make it easy to find what you are looking for.

The second table is first sorted into the five colour categories. The green category at the top is then sorted into food groups like the first table to make it especially easy to identify the foods you want to eat most of.

The remaining categories are then sorted alphabetically on food names.

The green category are the foods I live on.

The yellow category are foods I am more careful about eating and only in small amounts.

The orange category are foods I only eat rarely and in very small amounts.

The red category are things I avoid entirely.

I have grouped all drinks containing alcohol in the purple category although there are few or no carbohydrates in most of them. This is because alcohol can have an effect on insulin secretion similar to carbs, causing insulin levels to rise and block the release of fat for use as energy, and thereby weight loss.

That is clearly how my body works, but this may be another point where we aren't all the same and you may want to check how it works for you. This is where daily weight records come in handy. If you see your weight loss slowing or stopping if you drink alcohol, you'll probably have to go on the wagon like I did.

Or you could experiment and see if it's a temporary effect and the weight loss starts again after a bit. Entirely up to you. It's *your* fat handle, and you decide how to use it.

Product Name	Carbs Per 100g/ml	Product Name	Carbs Per 100g/ml
- CHEESE -		Milk, chocolate	11.2
Cheese spread	4.4	Milk, goats	4.4
Cheese, blue	2.4	Milk, semi skimmed	5.0
Cheese, cheddar	1.3	Milk, skimmed	5.0
Cheese, cottage	2.1	Milk, soya	0.8
Cheese, cottage, low-fat	4.0	Milk, whole	4.8
Cheese, cream	6.7	Milkshake, thick	20.0
Cheese, Feta	1.5	Yogurt, fruit	18.9
Cheese, hard and brie types	0.0	Yogurt, plain	6.2
Cheese, mozzarella	3.6	**- DRINKS -**	
Cheese, parmesan	4.0	Apple juice, unsweetened	10.2
Cheese, provolone	2.1	Bournvita, semi-skim milk	7.8
Cheese, ricotta	4.0	Bovril	2.9
Cheese, Swiss	2.1	Chocolate, Cadbury Instant Drink	66.8
- CONDIMENTS -		Coca-Cola	10.5
Blue cheese dressing	3.3	Cocoa, Cadbury	10.5
Brown sauce, No Frills	20.3	Cocoa, semi-skim milk	7.0
Fruity sauce, HP	31.0	Coffee	0.0
Gravy	5.0	Coffeemate	57.3
Horseradish sauce	17.9	Cranberry juice	13.4
Ketchup	26.7	Creamer	75.0
Marmite	1.8	Drinking chocolate, Semi skim	10.8
Mayonnaise, full fat	1.3	Fizzy drink, diet	0.1
Mint sauce	18.5	Fizzy drink, sweet	11.0
Mustard, smooth	9.7	Grape juice	12.4
Mustard, wholegrain	4.2	Grapefruit juice, unsweetened	8.3
Pickle	3.1	Horlicks + semi-skim milk	12.9
Salad cream	16.7	Horlicks, instant, water	10.1
Salt	0.0	Horlicks, low fat, inst, water	72.9
Sauce, brown HP	27.1	Lemon juice	8.3
Sauce, tomato ketchup, Heinz	24.7	Lemon juice, unsweetened	1.6
Soy sauce	8.3	Lemonade	8.9
Taramasalata	4.1	Lucozade	18.0
Tomato sauce	21.7	Orange juice	11.2
Vinegar	0.0	Orange juice, unsweetened	8.8
- DAIRY -		Ovaltine w/milk	13.0
Buttermilk	4.9	Pineapple juice, unsweet	10.5
Cream	3.3	Squash, orange	28.5
Cream, clotted	2.3	Tea	0.0
Cream, double	2.7	Tomato juice	3.7
Cream, single	4.1	Water	0.0
Cream, sour	4.0	**- FAT -**	
Cream, soured	3.8	Butter	0.0
Cream, whipping	2.8	Lard	0.0
Fromage frais	5.7	Margarine	0.0

Product Name	Carbs Per 100g/ml	Product Name	Carbs Per 100g/ml
Oils (all types)	0.0	Blueberries, sweetened	21.7
Shortening	0.0	Cantaloupe	8.1
Suet	12.1	Cherries, glaced	66.4
Treacle	67.2	Cherries, raw	10.9
- FISH -		Cherries, tin, syrup	18.4
Clams	4.7	Clementines, no skin	8.7
Cod in batter	7.5	Coconut, creamed, block	7.0
Cod steaks, in butter sauce, Birds Eye	3.9	Coconut, desiccated	6.4
Cod, fillet	0.0	Coconut, dried & sweetened	33.3
Crab	0.0	Currants	67.8
Fish cakes	15.1	Damsons, raw, stoned	8.6
Fish fingers	17.2	Dates, dried	76.0
Fish sticks, breaded	21.1	Dates, raw with stone	26.9
Fish, boiled or fried	0.0	Figs, dried	54.6
Haddock, fillet	0.0	Gooseberries	3.0
Herring, raw, smoked or fried	0.0	Grapefruit	10.6
Herring, marinated	19.0	Grapefruit, raw with skin	4.6
Lobster	0.0	Grapes	15.4
Mackerel in oil or brine	0.0	Honeydew melon	8.8
Mackerel in tomato sauce	1.8	Kiwi	14.5
Oysters	2.4	Kiwi fruit, no skin	10.6
Salmon	0.0	Lemon curd	62.7
Sardines, tin, tomato sauce	0.7	Lemon, with skin	3.2
Shrimp	0.0	Lychees, raw	14.3
Shrimp, breaded & fried	11.1	Mandarins, tin in juice	7.7
Trout	0.0	Mandarins, tin in syrup	13.4
Tuna	0.0	Mangoes, raw no stone or skin	14.1
- FRUIT -		Mangoes, tin in syrup	13.4
Apple	11.8	Melon, cantaloupe	4.2
Apple, dried	65.6	Melon, honeydew	6.6
Apple, no skin	12.7	Melon, water	7.1
Apples, cooking, raw, peeled	8.9	Nectarines	10.3
Applesauce, sweetened	17.6	Oranges	8.5
Applesauce, unsweetened	11.5	Papaya	10.9
Apricot, dried	61.1	Passion fruit	5.8
Apricot, raw	11.4	Paw paw	8.8
Apricot, semi-dried	36.5	Peach, raw	7.6
Apricot, stoned, raw	8.5	Peach, tin in juice	9.7
Apricot, tin, syrup	16.1	Peach, tin in syrup	14.0
Banana	22.9	Pear, in juice	10.5
Blackberries	11.7	Pear, in syrup	15.9
Blackcurrants	6.6	Pear, raw	10.0
Blackcurrants, tin, syrup	18.4	Peel, mixed dried	59.1
Blueberries	8.7	Pineapple, raw no skin	10.1

Product Name	Carbs Per 100g/ml	Product Name	Carbs Per 100g/ml
Pineapple, tin in juice	12.2	Flour, soya, full fat	23.5
Pineapple, tin in syrup	16.5	Flour, soya, low-fat	28.2
Plantain, boiled	28.5	Flour, wheat, brown	68.5
Plum, raw	8.3	Flour, wheat, white	77.7
Plum, tin in syrup	15.5	Flour, wheat, wholemeal	63.9
Prunes, semi-dry	34.0	Frosties	93.7
Prunes, tin in syrup	16.5	Lasagna	12.8
Raisins	74.4	Macaroni cheese	13.6
Raspberries, raw	6.9	Macaroni, cooked	30.7
Raspberries, tin in syrup	7.6	Macaroni, raw	75.8
Satsuma, raw	8.5	Muffin	40.4
Strawberries	7.2	Noodles, egg	70.1
Strawberries, tin in syrup	16.9	Oat bran	66.7
Tangerine	9.7	Oats, porridge, raw	60.0
- GRAIN -		Pancake	32.9
All-Bran	46.6	Pasta	69.1
Bagel	53.1	Pasta twists	51.8
Banana bread	55.0	Pita bread	55.0
Barley, cooked	27.8	Pizza	24.1
Biscuits	62.2	Popcorn	75.0
Bran flakes	69.3	Porridge, made with milk	13.7
Bran, wheat	26.8	Porridge, made with water	9.0
Bread, brown	44.3	Ready Brek	58.8
Bread, dinner roll	53.6	Rice krispies	89.7
Bread, hamburger bun	51.2	Rice, boiled	30.9
Bread, hotdog bun	51.2	Rice, brown cooked	23.1
Bread, med sliced white Kingsmill	44.1	Rice, long grain, white, frozen	27.1
Bread, white	49.3	Rice, raw	85.8
Bread, wholemeal Hovis	36.6	Rice, white cooked	27.8
Bulgur, cooked	18.7	Sesame seed	0.9
Buns, hot cross	58.5	Shortbread	63.9
Cereal, Alpen, no added sugar	61.3	Shredded wheat	68.3
Cereal, Bran Flakes, Kelloggs	66.0	Spaghetti	28.6
Cereal, Cheerios	75.9	Spaghetti, tinned	14.1
Cereals, unspecified	71.4	Special K	81.7
Chapati	48.3	Sunflower seed	18.6
Cornbread	48.3	Tortilla	60.9
Cornflakes	88.6	Waffle	33.3
Cornflakes, Crunchy Nut	93.7	Weetabix	75.7
Couscous, cooked	22.9	**- MEAT -**	
Crispbread, Ryvita Original	63.3	Bacon	0.5
Croissant	42.0	Beef	0.0
Croutons	60.0	Black pudding, fried	15.0
English muffin	43.9	Bologna	5.3
Flour, self raising	68.8	Bolognese sauce, Dolmio Original	10.3

Product Name	Carbs Per 100g/ml	Product Name	Carbs Per 100g/ml
Chicken, battered & fried	8.3	Peanuts, plain	12.5
Chicken, flour & fried	1.6	Pecan nuts	4.0
Chicken, hot & spicy wings	5.4	Pine nuts	9.4
Chicken, meat only	0.0	Pistachios	17.7
Duck	0.0	Walnut	7.5
Corned beef	0.8	**- SWEETS -**	
Dumplings	24.5	Angelfood cake	58.0
Egg, raw	0.6	Brownie	64.3
Frankfurters	3.0	Cake	65.6
Goose	0.0	Cake, pound	55.4
Ham	2.6	Cake, rich fruit, iced	62.7
Ham, honey roast	2.4	Cake, snack	65.1
Ham, smoked	0.8	Cakes, rich fruit	59.6
Hotdog	3.4	Cereal bar, Cherry Nutrigrain	69.0
Lamb	0.0	Cheesecake	25.0
Liver paté	2.5	Cheeselets	56.9
Liver paté, low fat	4.9	Choc. chip cookie, homemade	56.3
Liver sausage	4.3	Chocolate syrup	63.2
Luncheon meat, tin	5.5	Chocolate, milk	57.0
Marrow, raw	2.2	Chocolate, dark	54.0
Peperami	1.7	Cookie, oatmeal	86.7
Polony	14.2	Cookie, peanut butter	70.0
Pork	0.0	Cookie, sugar	60.0
Pork ribs, Chinese style sauce	6.9	Crackers, Cream	68.3
Quorn	2.0	Crust, pie	56.3
Ratatouille	3.0	Custard	16.6
Ravioli	10.3	Danish pastry	51.3
Salami	1.9	Digestive biscuits	67.0
Sausages, pork	10.4	Doughnuts	50.7
Soup, chicken	4.4	Eccles cakes	59.3
Soup, oxtail	6.7	Eclairs	26.1
Stuffing, parsley/thyme/lemon, cooked	28.4	Fruit cocktail in juice	7.2
Stuffing, sage/onion, cooked	23.0	Fruit cocktail in syrup	14.8
Turkey	0.0	Fudge	63.2
Veal	0.0	Graham cracker	78.6
- NUTS -		Honey	82.0
Almonds	9.8	Ice cream	25.8
Brazil nut	3.1	Ice-cream, Choc ice	28.1
Cashews	28.9	Ice-cream, lemon sorbet	34.2
Chestnuts	36.6	Ice-cream, vanilla	24.4
Hazelnuts	6.0	Jaffa cakes	67.8
Macadamia nuts	5.2	Jam tart	62.0
Peanut butter	16.0	Jam, blackcurrant	60.5
Peanuts, dry roasted	10.3	Jam, fruit	69.0

Product Name	Carbs Per 100g/ml	Product Name	Carbs Per 100g/ml
Jam/Jelly	65.0	Beans, broad	11.7
Kit Kat	64.3	Beans, butter	13.0
m&m's, peanut	60.0	Beans, French	4.7
m&m's, plain	71.4	Beans, kidney	22.5
Marshmallows	82.0	Beans, mung	15.3
Marzipan	50.2	Beans, red kidney	17.8
Meringue with cream	40.0	Beans, runner	2.3
Milky Way	70.5	Beans, soya	5.1
Mince pie	59.0	Beans, white, canned	21.4
Mincemeat	62.1	Bean sprouts	2.5
Pastry	42.3	Beetroot, boiled	9.5
Pie, apple	31.3	Beetroot, pickled	11.2
Pie, blueberry	30.6	Broccoli, cooked	3.9
Pie, cherry	32.5	Broccoli, raw	2.9
Pie, chocolate	33.6	Brussels sprouts	5.5
Pie, coconut	29.8	Cabbage, white, boiled	2.5
Pie, lemon meringue	46.9	Cabbage, white or red, raw	4.9
Pie, pecan	53.7	Carrots, old, boiled	4.9
Pie, pumpkin	25.8	Carrots, old, raw	2.5
Pudding, hot crunch banana	75.0	Carrots, tinned	4.2
Pudding, rice	15.4	Carrots, young boiled	4.4
Pudding, sponge	45.3	Carrots, young raw	5.9
Reece's Peanut Butter Cups	55.6	Cauliflower, raw	2.2
Snickers	61.4	Celery, raw	3.3
Sugar, brown	93.8	Chickpeas	19.0
Sugar, demerara	100.0	Chicory, raw	2.8
Sugar, granulated	95.2	Corn on the cob	22.2
Sugar, powdered	100.0	Corn, canned	18.5
Sugar, white	100.0	Corn, frozen	20.4
Syrup	79.0	Courgette, raw	1.8
Syrup, maple	65.0	Crisps, cheese & onion flavour	48.5
Yogurt, frozen	25.0	Cucumber	1.5
- VEGETABLES -		Cucumber, pickled	16.1
Artichoke	11.7	Curly kale, raw	1.4
Asparagus, raw	2.8	Eggplant	9.1
Asparagus, tin	1.4	Fennel, raw	1.8
Aubergine	2.8	Garlic, raw	16.3
Avocado	6.5	Gherkin, pickled	2.6
Bamboo shoots	9.7	Gourd, raw	0.8
Beans, aduki	22.5	Kale, cooked	6.2
Beans, baked Heinz	13.6	Leeks, boiled	2.6
Beans, baked, canned	18.9	Leeks, raw	2.9
Beans, black, cooked	23.3	Lentils, boiled	16.9

Product Name	Carbs Per 100g/ml	Product Name	Carbs Per 100g/ml
Lentils, red	17.5	Squash, summer, cooked	4.4
Lettuce	2.7	Squash, summer, raw	2.3
Lima beans	28.3	Swede, boiled	2.3
Lime juice	10.5	Sweet potato, boiled	20.5
Mixed veg, frozen, boiled	6.6	Sweetcorn baby, canned	2.0
Mushrooms, raw	1.7	Sweetcorn kernels, canned	26.6
Okra, cooked	6.3	Sweetcorn on cob, whole	11.6
Okra, raw	3.0	Tofu, soya bean	2.0
Olives	4.5	Tomato	2.5
Onion, cooked	7.7	Tomato puree	16.0
Onion, raw	7.9	Tomato, canned with juice	3.0
Onions, cocktail	3.1	Tomato, chopped, tinned	5.7
Onions, fried	14.1	Turnip	2.0
Onions, pickled	5.8	Vegetables, Chinese, frozen	7.2
Parsnip, raw	10.1	Watercress	0.4
Peas, canned	13.5	- ALCOHOL -	
Peas, frozen, boiled	9.7	Ale, brown	3.0
Peas, mange-tout	3.5	Ale, strong	6.1
Peas, mushy	13.8	Beer	3.7
Peas, petit-pois, frozen, boiled	5.5	Beer, bitter, tin	2.3
Peas, processed	17.5	Beer, light	1.7
Peas, raw	5.8	Brandy	0.0
Peppers, green	2.6	Cider, dry	2.6
Peppers, red	6.4	Cider, sweet	4.3
Potato salad	11.2	Cognac, Armagnac	0.0
Potato, boiled	17.0	Daiquiri	6.7
Potato, frying chips frozen	30.3	Dessert wine	12.6
Potato, hash browns	56.3	Gin	0.0
Potato, mashed	17.1	Lager	1.5
Potato, roast	25.9	Port	12.0
Pumpkin	2.2	Rum	0.0
Radish	1.9	Sherry, dry	1.7
Rhubarb, raw	3.0	Sherry, sweet	6.7
Rhubarb, tin in syrup	16.9	Stout	4.2
Saveloy	10.1	Table wine	2.9
Snap Beans	0.0	Vodka	0.0
Soup, tomato	8.4	Whisky	0.0
Soup, vegetable	8.4	Wine, red	0.3
Spinach, boiled	0.8	Wine, rosé	2.5
Spinach, raw	3.3	Wine, white, dry	0.6
Spring greens	1.6	Wine, white, med	3.4
Spring onions	1.6	Wine, white, sweet	5.9

Product Name	Carbs Per 100g/ml	Product Name	Carbs Per 100g/ml
- CHEESE -	**0 - 4.9**	**- FAT -**	
Cheese spread	4.4	Butter	0.0
Cheese, blue	2.4	Lard	0.0
Cheese, cheddar	1.3	Margarine	0.0
Cheese, cottage	2.1	Oils (all types)	0.0
Cheese, cottage, low-fat	4.0	Shortening	0.0
Cheese, Feta	1.5	**- FISH -**	
Cheese, hard and brie types	0.0	Clams	4.7
Cheese, mozzarella	3.6	Cod steaks, in butter sauce, Birds Eye	3.9
Cheese, parmesan	4.0	Cod, fillet	0.0
Cheese, provolone	2.1	Crab	0.0
Cheese, ricotta	4.0	Fish, boiled or fried	0.0
Cheese, Swiss	2.1	Haddock, fillet	0.0
- CONDIMENTS -		Herring, raw, smoked or fried	0.0
Blue cheese dressing	3.3	Lobster	0.0
Marmite	1.8	Mackerel in oil or brine	0.0
Mayonnaise, full fat	1.3	Mackerel in tomato sauce	1.8
Mustard, wholegrain	4.2	Oysters	2.4
Pickle	3.1	Salmon	0.0
Salt	0.0	Sardines, tin, tomato sauce	0.7
Taramasalata	4.1	Shrimp	0.0
Vinegar	0.0	Trout	0.0
- DAIRY -		Tuna	0.0
Buttermilk	4.9	**- FRUIT -**	
Cream	3.3	Gooseberries	3.0
Cream, clotted	2.3	Grapefruit, raw with skin	4.6
Cream, double	2.7	Lemon, with skin	3.2
Cream, single	4.1	Melon, cantaloupe	4.2
Cream, sour	4.0	**- GRAIN -**	
Cream, soured	3.8	Sesame seed	0.9
Cream, whipping	2.8	**- MEAT -**	
Milk, goats	4.4	Bacon	0.5
Milk, soya	0.8	Beef	0.0
Milk, whole	4.8	Chicken, flour & fried	1.6
- DRINKS -		Chicken, meat only	0.0
Bovril	2.9	Corned beef	0.8
Coffee	0.0	Duck	0.0
Fizzy drink, diet	0.1	Egg, raw	0.6
Lemon juice, unsweetened	1.6	Frankfurters	3.0
Tea	0.0	Goose	0.0
Tomato juice	3.7	Ham	2.6
Water	0.0	Ham, honey roast	2.4
		Ham, smoked	0.8
		Hotdog	3.4

Product Name	Carbs Per 100g/ml	Product Name	Carbs Per 100g/ml
Lamb	0.0	Onions, cocktail	3.1
Liver paté	2.5	Peas, mange-tout	3.5
Liver paté, low fat	4.9	Peppers, green	2.6
Liver sausage	4.3	Pumpkin	2.2
Marrow, raw	2.2	Radish	1.9
Pepperoni	1.7	Rhubarb, raw	3.0
Pork	0.0	Snap Beans	0.0
Quorn	2.0	Spinach, boiled	0.8
Ratatouille	3.0	Spinach, raw	3.3
Salami	1.9	Spring greens	1.6
Soup, chicken	4.4	Spring onions	1.6
Turkey	0.0	Squash, summer, cooked	4.4
Veal	0.0	Squash, summer, raw	2.3
- NUTS -		Swede, boiled	2.3
Brazil nut	3.1	Sweetcorn baby, canned	2.0
Pecan nuts	4.0	Tofu, soya bean	2.0
- VEGETABLES -		Tomato	2.5
Asparagus, raw	2.8	Tomato, canned with juice	3.0
Asparagus, tin	1.4	Turnip	2.0
Aubergine	2.8	Watercress	0.4
Beans, French	4.7		**5 - 9.9**
Beans, runner	2.3	Almonds	9.8
Bean sprouts	2.5	Apples, cooking, raw, peeled	8.9
Broccoli, cooked	3.9	Apricot, stoned, raw	8.5
Broccoli, raw	2.9	Avocado	6.5
Cabbage, white or red, raw	4.9	Bamboo shoots	9.7
Cabbage, white, boiled	2.5	Beans, soya	5.1
Carrots, old, boiled	4.9	Beetroot, boiled	9.5
Carrots, old, raw	2.5	Blackcurrants	6.6
Carrots, tinned	4.2	Blueberries	8.7
Carrots, young boiled	4.4	Bologna	5.3
Cauliflower, raw	2.2	Bournvita, semi-skim milk	7.8
Celery, raw	3.3	Brussels sprouts	5.5
Chicory, raw	2.8	Cantaloupe	8.1
Courgette, raw	1.8	Carrots, young raw	5.9
Cucumber	1.5	Cheese, cream	6.7
Curly kale, raw	1.4	Chicken, battered & fried	8.3
Fennel, raw	1.8	Chicken, hot & spicy wings	5.4
Gherkin, pickled	2.6	Clementines, no skin	8.7
Gourd, raw	0.8	Cocoa, semi-skim milk	7.0
Leeks, boiled	2.6	Coconut, creamed, block	7.0
Leeks, raw	2.9	Coconut, desiccated	6.4
Lettuce	2.7	Cod in batter	7.5
Mushrooms, raw	1.7	Damsons, raw, stoned	8.6
Okra, raw	3.0	Eggplant	9.1
Olives	4.5	Fromage frais	5.7

Product Name	Carbs Per 100g/ml	Product Name	Carbs Per 100g/ml
Fruit cocktail in juice	7.2	Walnut	7.5
Grapefruit juice, unsweetened	8.3	Yogurt, plain	6.2
Gravy	5.0		10 - 19.9
Hazelnuts	6.0	Apple	11.8
Honeydew melon	8.8	Apple juice, unsweetened	10.2
Kale, cooked	6.2	Apple, no skin	12.7
Lemon juice	8.3	Applesauce, sweetened	17.6
Lemonade	8.9	Applesauce, unsweetened	11.5
Luncheon meat, tin	5.5	Apricot, raw	11.4
Macadamia nuts	5.2	Apricot, tin, syrup	16.1
Mandarins, tin in juice	7.7	Artichoke	11.7
Melon, honeydew	6.6	Beans, baked Heinz	13.6
Melon, water	7.1	Beans, baked, canned	18.9
Milk, semi skimmed	5.0	Beans, broad	11.7
Milk, skimmed	5.0	Beans, butter	13.0
Mixed veg, frozen, boiled	6.6	Beans, mung	15.3
Mustard, smooth	9.7	Beans, red kidney	17.8
Okra, cooked	6.3	Beetroot, pickled	11.2
Onion, cooked	7.7	Black pudding, fried	15.0
Onion, raw	7.9	Blackberries	11.7
Onions, pickled	5.8	Blackcurrants, tin, syrup	18.4
Orange juice, unsweetened	8.8	Bolognese sauce, Dolmio Original	10.3
Oranges	8.5	Bulgur, cooked	18.7
Passion fruit	5.8	Cherries, raw	10.9
Paw paw	8.8	Cherries, tin, syrup	18.4
Peach, raw	7.6	Chickpeas	19.0
Peach, tin in juice	9.7	Coca-Cola	10.5
Peas, frozen, boiled	9.7	Cocoa, Cadbury	10.5
Peas, petit-pois, frozen, boiled	5.5	Corn, canned	18.5
Peas, raw	5.8	Cranberry juice	13.4
Peppers, red	6.4	Cucumber, pickled	16.1
Pine nuts	9.4	Custard	16.6
Plum, raw	8.3	Drinking chocolate, Semi skim	10.8
Pork ribs, Chinese style sauce	6.9	Fish cakes	15.1
Porridge, made with water	9.0	Fish fingers	17.2
Raspberries, raw	6.9	Fizzy drink, sweet	11.0
Raspberries, tin in syrup	7.6	Fruit cocktail in syrup	14.8
Satsuma, raw	8.5	Garlic, raw	16.3
Soup, oxtail	6.7	Grape juice	12.4
Soup, tomato	8.4	Grapefruit	10.6
Soup, vegetable	8.4	Grapes	15.4
Soy sauce	8.3	Herring, marinated	19.0
Strawberries	7.2	Horlicks + semi-skim milk	12.9
Tangerine	9.7	Horlicks, instant, water	10.1
Tomato, chopped, tinned	5.7	Horseradish sauce	17.9
Vegetables, Chinese, frozen	7.2	Kiwi	14.5

Product Name	Carbs Per 100g/ml	Product Name	Carbs Per 100g/ml
Kiwi fruit, no skin	10.6	Sausages, pork	10.4
Lasagna	12.8	Saveloy	10.1
Lentils, boiled	16.9	Shrimp, breaded & fried	11.1
Lentils, red	17.5	Spaghetti, tinned	14.1
Lime juice	10.5	Strawberries, tin in syrup	16.9
Lucozade	18.0	Suet	12.1
Lychees, raw	14.3	Sunflower seed	18.6
Macaroni cheese	13.6	Sweetcorn on cob, whole	11.6
Mandarins, tin in syrup	13.4	Tomato puree	16.0
Mangoes, raw no stone or skin	14.1	Yogurt, fruit	18.9
Mangoes, tin in syrup	13.4		> 20
Milk, chocolate	11.2	All-Bran	46.6
Mint sauce	18.5	Angelfood cake	58.0
Nectarines	10.3	Apple, dried	65.6
Onions, fried	14.1	Apricot, dried	61.1
Orange juice	11.2	Apricot, semi-dried	36.5
Ovaltine w/milk	13.0	Bagel	53.1
Papaya	10.9	Banana	22.9
Parsnip, raw	10.1	Banana bread	55.0
Peach, tin in syrup	14.0	Barley, cooked	27.8
Peanut butter	16.0	Beans, aduki	22.5
Peanuts, dry roasted	10.3	Beans, black, cooked	23.3
Peanuts, plain	12.5	Beans, kidney	22.5
Pear, in juice	10.5	Beans, white, canned	21.4
Pear, in syrup	15.9	Biscuits	62.2
Pear, raw	10.0	Blueberries, sweetened	21.7
Peas, canned	13.5	Bran flakes	69.3
Peas, mushy	13.8	Bran, wheat	26.8
Peas, processed	17.5	Bread, brown	44.3
Pineapple juice, unsweet	10.5	Bread, dinner roll	53.6
Pineapple, raw no skin	10.1	Bread, hamburger bun	51.2
Pineapple, tin in juice	12.2	Bread, hotdog bun	51.2
Pineapple, tin in syrup	16.5	Bread, med sliced white Kingsmill	44.1
Pistachios	17.7	Bread, white	49.3
Plum, tin in syrup	15.5	Bread, wholemeal Hovis	36.6
Polony	14.2	Brown sauce, No Frills	20.3
Porridge, made with milk	13.7	Brownie	64.3
Potato salad	11.2	Buns, hot cross	58.5
Potato, boiled	17.0	Cake	65.6
Potato, mashed	17.1	Cake, pound	55.4
Prunes, tin in syrup	16.5	Cake, rich fruit, iced	62.7
Pudding, rice	15.4	Cake, snack	65.1
Ravioli	10.3	Cakes, rich fruit	59.6
Rhubarb, tin in syrup	16.9	Cashews	28.9
Salad cream	16.7	Cereal bar, Cherry Nutrigrain	69.0

Product Name	Carbs Per 100g/ml	Product Name	Carbs Per 100g/ml
Cereal, Alpen, no added sugar	61.3	Flour, self raising	68.8
Cereal, Bran Flakes, Kelloggs	66.0	Flour, soya, full fat	23.5
Cereal, Cheerios	75.9	Flour, soya, low-fat	28.2
Cereals, unspecified	71.4	Flour, wheat, brown	68.5
Chapati	48.3	Flour, wheat, white	77.7
Cheesecake	25.0	Flour, wheat, wholemeal	63.9
Cheeselets	56.9	Frosties	93.7
Cherries, glaced	66.4	Fruity sauce, HP	31.0
Chestnuts	36.6	Fudge	63.2
Choc. chip cookie, homemade	56.3	Graham cracker	78.6
Chocolate syrup	63.2	Honey	82.0
Chocolate, Cadbury Instant Drink	66.8	Horlicks, low fat, inst, water	72.9
Chocolate, dark	54.0	Ice cream	25.8
Chocolate, milk	57.0	Ice-cream, Choc ice	28.1
Coconut, dried & sweetened	33.3	Ice-cream, lemon sorbet	34.2
Coffeemate	57.3	Ice-cream, vanilla	24.4
Cookie, oatmeal	86.7	Jaffa cakes	67.8
Cookie, peanut butter	70.0	Jam tart	62.0
Cookie, sugar	60.0	Jam, blackcurrant	60.5
Corn on the cob	22.2	Jam, fruit	69.0
Corn, frozen	20.4	Jam/Jelly	65.0
Cornbread	48.3	Ketchup	26.7
Cornflakes	88.6	Kit Kat	64.3
Cornflakes, Crunchy Nut	93.7	Lemon curd	62.7
Couscous, cooked	22.9	Lima beans	28.3
Crackers, Cream	68.3	m&m's, peanut	60.0
Creamer	75.0	m&m's, plain	71.4
Crispbread, Ryvita Original	63.3	Macaroni, cooked	30.7
Crisps, cheese & onion flavour	49.6	Macaroni, raw	75.8
Croissant	42.0	Marshmallows	82.0
Croutons	60.0	Marzipan	50.2
Crust, pie	56.3	Meringue with cream	40.0
Currants	67.8	Milkshake, thick	20.0
Danish pastry	51.3	Milky Way	70.5
Dates, dried	76.0	Mince pie	59.0
Dates, raw with stone	26.9	Mincemeat	62.1
Digestive biscuits	67.0	Muffin	40.4
Doughnuts	50.7	Noodles, egg	70.1
Dumplings	24.5	Oat bran	66.7
Eccles cakes	59.3	Oats, porridge, raw	60.0
Eclairs	26.1	Pancake	32.9
English muffin	43.9	Pasta	69.1
Figs, dried	54.6	Pasta twists	51.8
Fish sticks, breaded	21.1	Pastry	42.3

Product Name	Carbs Per 100g/ml	Product Name	Carbs Per 100g/ml
Peel, mixed dried	59.1	Sugar, granulated	95.2
Pie, apple	31.3	Sugar, powdered	100.0
Pie, blueberry	30.6	Sugar, white	100.0
Pie, cherry	32.5	Sweet potato, boiled	20.5
Pie, chocolate	33.6	Sweetcorn kernels, canned	26.6
Pie, coconut	29.8	Syrup	79.0
Pie, lemon meringue	46.9	Syrup, maple	65.0
Pie, pecan	53.7	Tomato sauce	21.7
Pie, pumpkin	25.8	Tortilla	60.9
Pita bread	55.0	Treacle	67.2
Pizza	24.1	Waffle	33.3
Plantain, boiled	28.5	Weetabix	75.7
Popcorn	75.0	Yogurt, frozen	25.0
Potato, frying chips frozen	30.3	**- ALCOHOL -**	
Potato, hash browns	56.3	Ale, brown	3.0
Potato, roast	25.9	Ale, strong	6.1
Prunes, semi-dry	34.0	Beer	3.7
Pudding, hot crunch banana	75.0	Beer, bitter, tin	2.3
Pudding, sponge	45.3	Beer, light	1.7
Raisins	74.4	Brandy	0.0
Ready Brek	58.8	Cider, dry	2.6
Reece's Peanut Butter Cups	55.6	Cider, sweet	4.3
Rice krispies	89.7	Cognac, Armagnac	0.0
Rice, boiled	30.9	Daiquiri	6.7
Rice, brown cooked	23.1	Dessert wine	12.6
Rice, long grain, white, frozen	27.1	Gin	0.0
Rice, raw	85.8	Lager	1.5
Rice, white cooked	27.8	Port	12.0
Sauce, brown HP	27.1	Rum	0.0
Sauce, tomato ketchup, Heinz	24.7	Sherry, dry	1.7
Shortbread	63.9	Sherry, sweet	6.7
Shredded wheat	68.3	Stout	4.2
Snickers	61.4	Table wine	2.9
Spaghetti	28.6	Vodka	0.0
Special K	81.7	Whisky	0.0
Squash, orange	28.5	Wine, red	0.3
Stuffing, parsley/thyme/lemon, cooked	28.4	Wine, rosé	2.5
Stuffing, sage/onion, cooked	23.0	Wine, white, dry	0.6
Sugar, brown	93.8	Wine, white, med	3.4
Sugar, demerara	100.0	Wine, white, sweet	5.9

6. Picture cookbook

What follows is not a conventional cookbook. I won't be giving you lists of ingredients or tell you how to cook, apart from a few personal pointers. This food is so simple and easy to cook it's not necessary. Anyway, I have always thought cooking was best based on using good ingredients and doing as little as possible to them so as not to ruin them, and this is no less true for no-carb cooking.

So I'll let my pictures of the food I am eating tell most of the story and add just a few comments in the hope that you will be inspired to cook and eat similar things.

Some people may think that the portions in the pictures aren't very large. Maybe, but remember that these pictures are of breakfasts, lunches and dinners, so some portions will be smaller and some larger.

Besides, these are the portion sizes that fill me. If they don't fill you, make them bigger without making them huge.

This is not a calorie restricted diet, but the simple fact is that protein and fat are more filling than carbohydrates, and fill for longer, so chances are that these portions will also satisfy you.

I didn't eat a lot more before I started eating no-carb, and I've been eating smaller portions than this on calorie restricted diets without losing much weight, so it's not the smaller portions that make me lose weight now, or at least not those alone.

Maybe it's these portion sizes in combination with the loss of carbs that do it for me, and this is something you should consider if you think you are not losing enough and you are eating significantly larger portions than shown here.

Bon appetit.

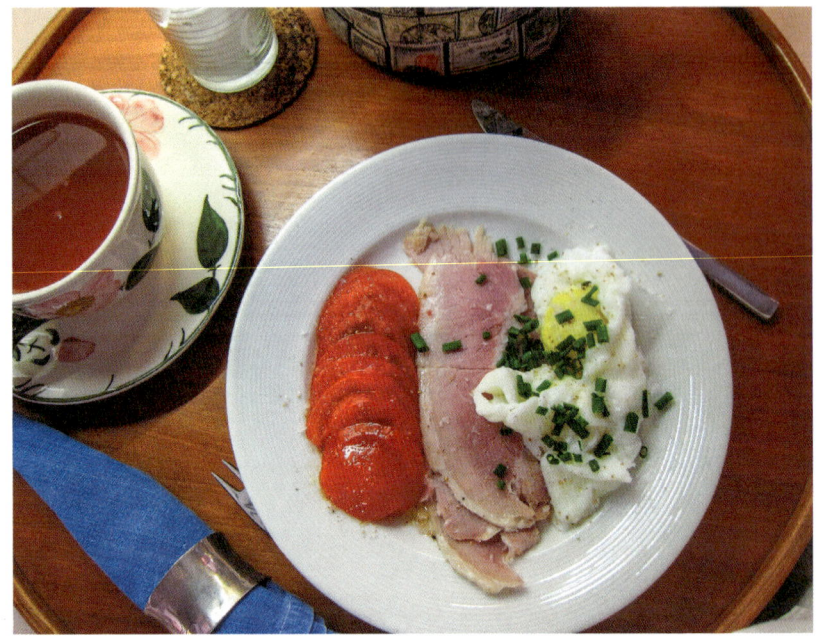

Ham, tomato with olive oil and poached egg with chives

A tasty, filling breakfast that easily keeps me going till lunch. I drink a pot of black tea with it, but coffee should be fine too. No sugar, and preferably no milk (use real cream for white coffee).

The glass at the top of the picture is full of ice cubes to cool my tea to a temperature I can drink, because it's too hot for me straight out of a freshly brewed pot. I thought I was the only person in the world who did this until one day at breakfast in a hotel restaurant I heard someone else order tea with a bowl of ice cubes.

A reminder that we're never alone :-)

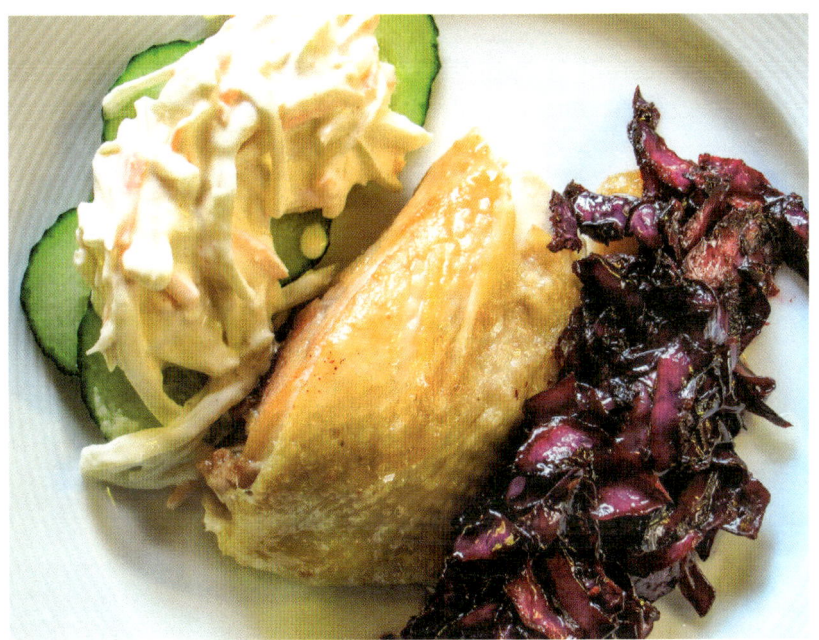

Chicken breast with red cabbage, coleslaw and cucumber

The chicken is cooked in its own juices in a slow cooker and the red cabbage is fried for 5 minutes in olive oil, with salt, white pepper and a tablespoon of vinegar added halfway.

The coleslaw is a low-carb version from my local deli, but read labels carefully as some coleslaws have a lot of added sugar.

The cucumber slices are raw.

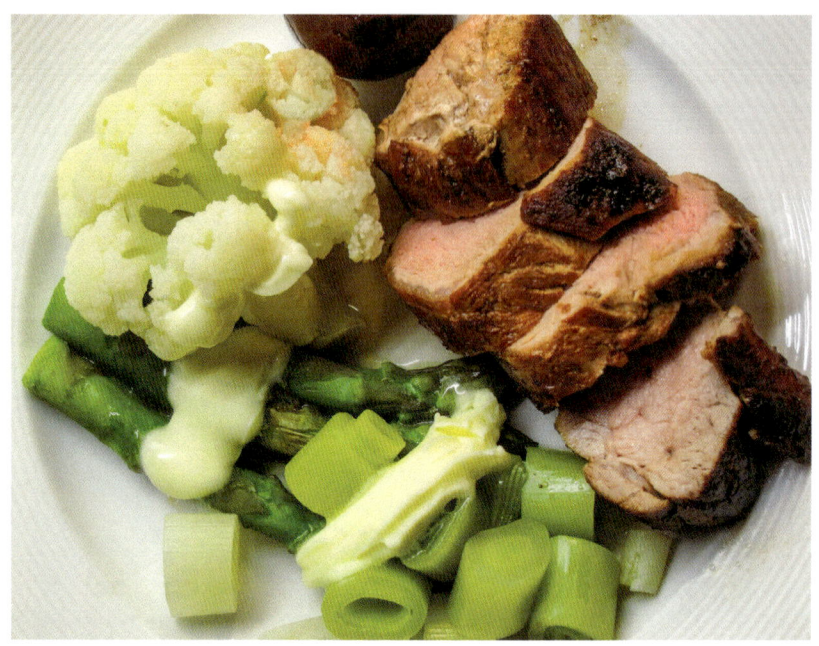

Pork tenderloin with cauliflower, asparagus, leeks and a knob of butter

The tenderloin pan fried in olive oil and the vegetables are boiled or steamed.

Be careful not to overcook them. Sad, soggy cooked-to-death vegetables are a likely reason so many people eat their veggies only as a chore. Cook them *al dente* and they will look, smell, feel and taste great, the way food should.

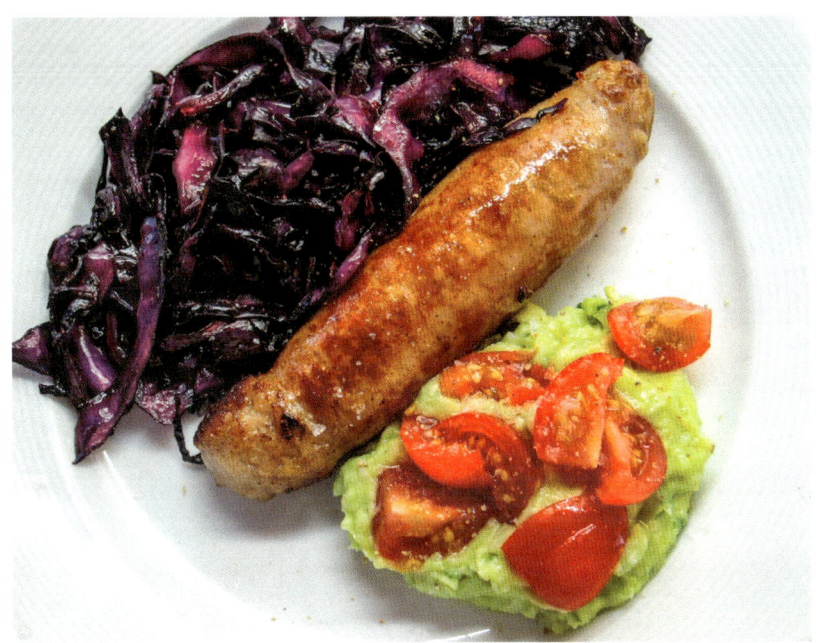

Pork sausage with red cabbage, creamed avocado and tomato

The sausage is from my local butcher and is made from local, free range pork (in fact, he rears the pigs himself). Be careful with sausages as some have lots of flour and other carbs added. Read the label or ask your butcher.

The red cabbage is fried for 5 minutes in olive oil, with salt, white pepper and a tablespoon of vinegar added halfway.

The creamed avocado is made by chopping a small avocado into cubes and whizzing those for ten seconds in a small food processor. Just a little salt and pepper added.

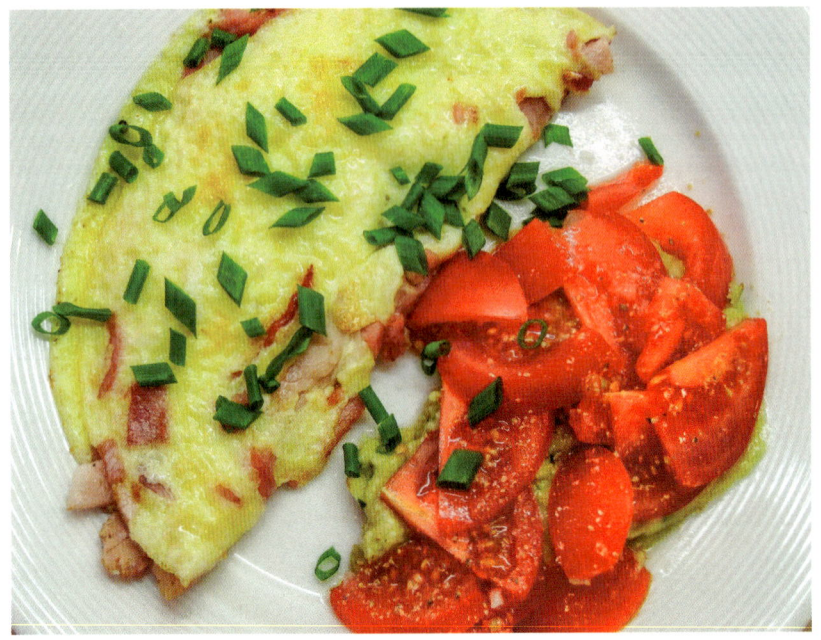

Ham omelette with creamed avocado, tomato and chives

This omelette is made from one medium size egg and a couple of chopped slices of ham.

I fry the ham in a little olive oil while I whisk the egg with about a tablespoon of double cream and a teaspoon of water (using one of the half eggshells as a measure to make things simple and keep down the washing-up). I like my omelettes slightly on the runny side, but of course you will cook yours to your own taste.

The creamed avocado is made from half an avocado chopped into cubes and whizzed for ten seconds in a small food processor.

Top off with chopped chives for taste, texture and colour.

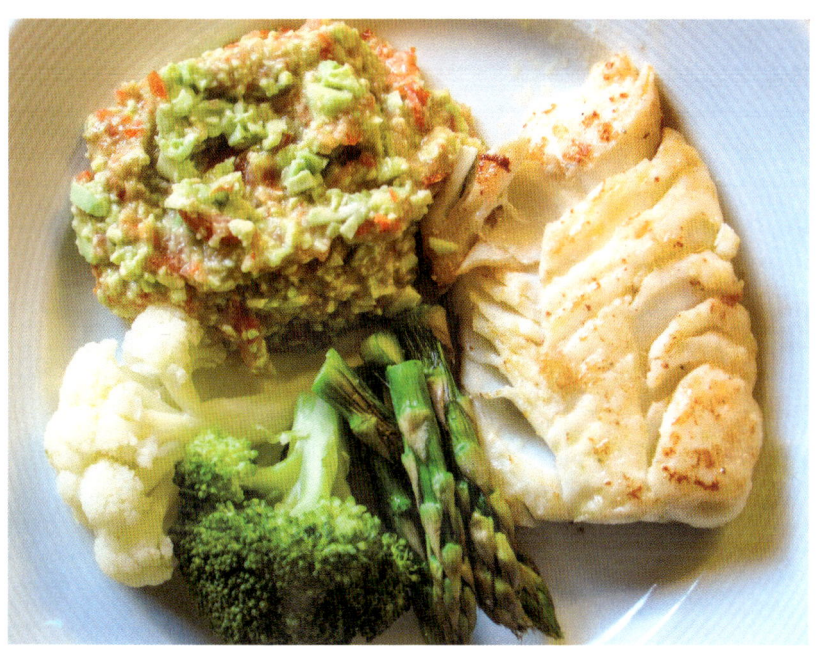

Pan fried cod with steamed vegetables and guacamole

The cod is lightly fried in olive oil until tender, and as always with vegetables, I am careful not to overcook them.

I call the accompaniment guacamole, but it isn't really. Guacamole takes a long time to make and needs a lot of things that I don't normally have, so this is my own take on it:

I cube half an avocado, a piece of cucumber and a tomato, then whizz that mix for a few seconds in a small food processor. If you want the bite of real guacamole, add a pinch of chili, but I don't so I just add salt, white pepper and maybe some garlic.

It takes 20-30 minutes to make real guacamole. This takes 2.

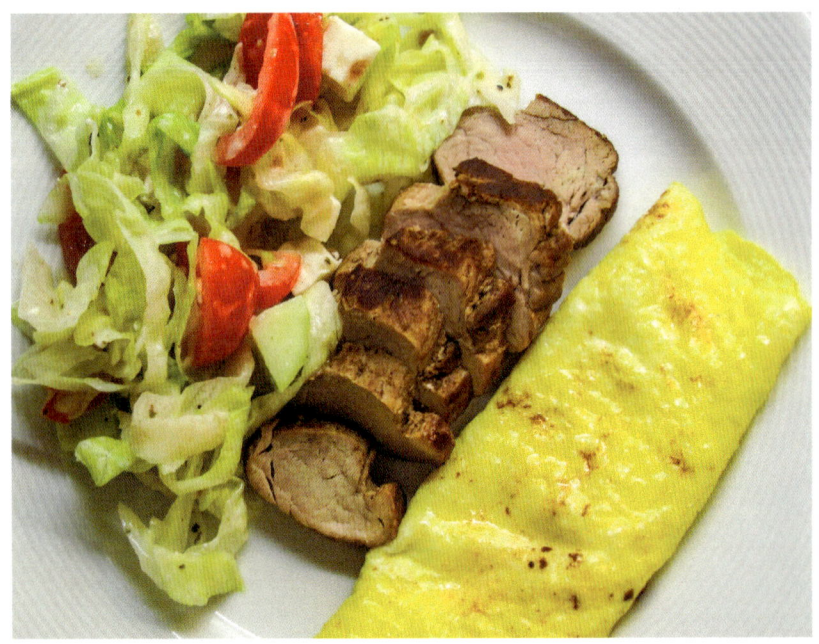

Pork tenderloin with plain omelette, green salad and tomato

I pan fry the tenderloin whole in olive oil, or a mix of olive oil and butter, and leave it to rest for a few minutes before slicing it.

The omelette is made from one egg whisked with a tablespoon of cream and a teaspoon of water.

This salad is made from lettuce, avocado, Feta cheese and tomatoes, with a simple oil and vinegar dressing. Use any dressing you like as long as you don't smother the salad in dressing, or if you do make sure it's low carb.

As always - read the label of anything you don't make yourself from raw materials.

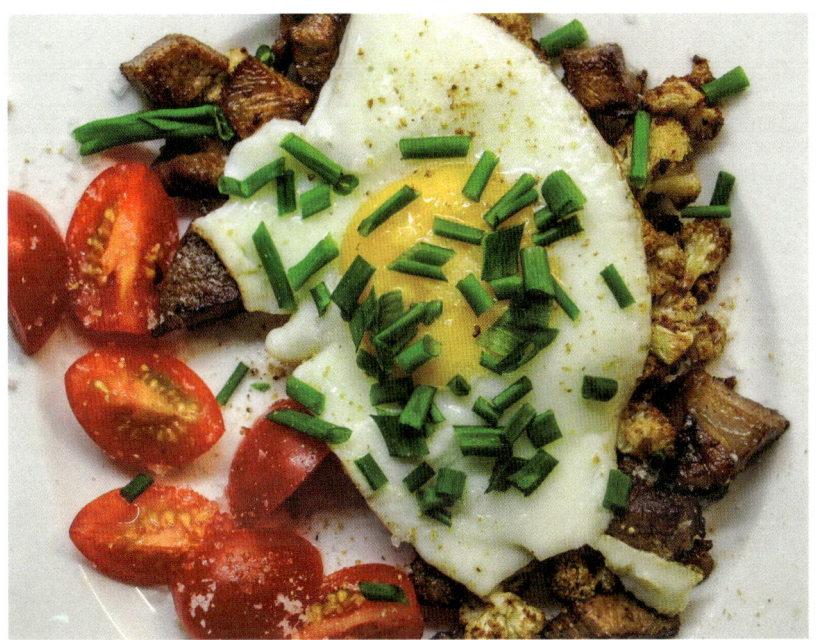

Hash with fried egg, tomatoes and chives

I make the hash with whatever was left over from last night—pork, chicken or beef and whatever vegetables I had with it, this time cauliflower—sometimes with a little sliced onion, but absolutely none of the potatoes that normally belong in hash.

Add a fried egg and a tomato or two and top off with chives.

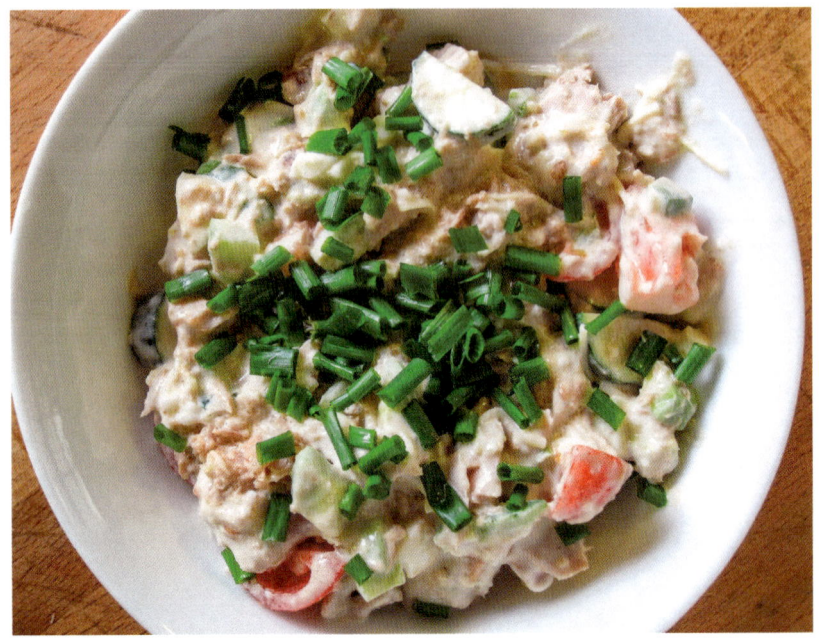

Tuna salad with chives

One way to make it easy to eat no-carb for lunch. In this salad I take a tin of tuna (in oil or in brine as you prefer) and mix it with coarsely chopped tomato, cucumber and avocado.

I drain off the tin dressing and make my own salad dressing from two tablespoons of yoghurt and a tablespoon of crème fraiche. I mix it all together and season with salt and white pepper and top it off with whatever tasty greenery I have to hand, in this case chives.

This takes a few minutes to make in the morning, or even the night before, and keeps fine until lunch if you can keep it cool. If not, keep the tuna in the tin and simply mix it in with the rest just before lunch.

This delicious no-carb lunch fits neatly into any plastic box with a tight fitting lid so you can take it anywhere you need.

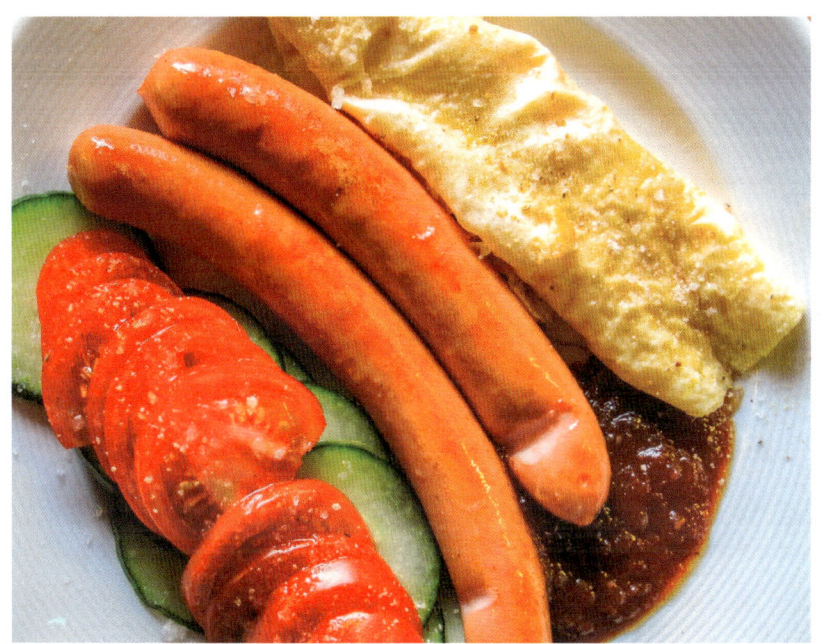

Frankfurters with omelette, tomatoes, cucumber and ketchup

Some frankfurters are full of flour, but these are low carb. As always with anything you don't cook from raw ingredients, read the label carefully and avoid anything with high carbohydrate contents.

The omelette is made from one egg whisked with a tablespoon of cream and a teaspoon of water.

The ketchup is home made and therefore low carb, but even if you don't make your own, a small dollop like this of the commercial stuff only contains a gram or so of carbs. With condiments it's not so much the content per 100 g that's meaningful but the amount you use of it.

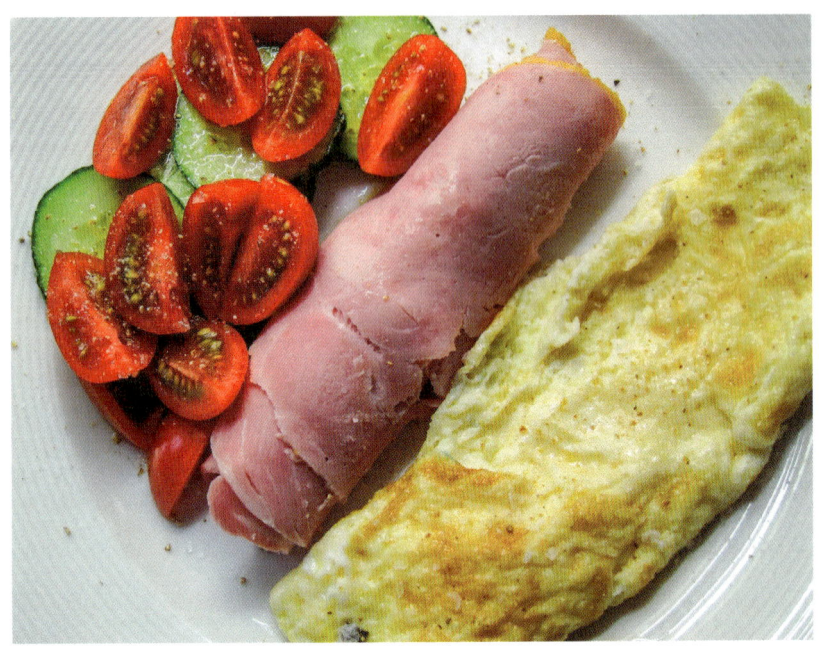

Ham with omelette, tomato and cucumber

A couple of slices of ham and an omelette made from one egg whisked with a tablespoon of cream and a teaspoon of water.

The ham can be cold or you can warm it on the same pan you use for the omelette.

The tomatoes and cucumber are raw with just salt, white pepper and a little olive oil.

This is my favourite breakfast but works just as well for lunch.

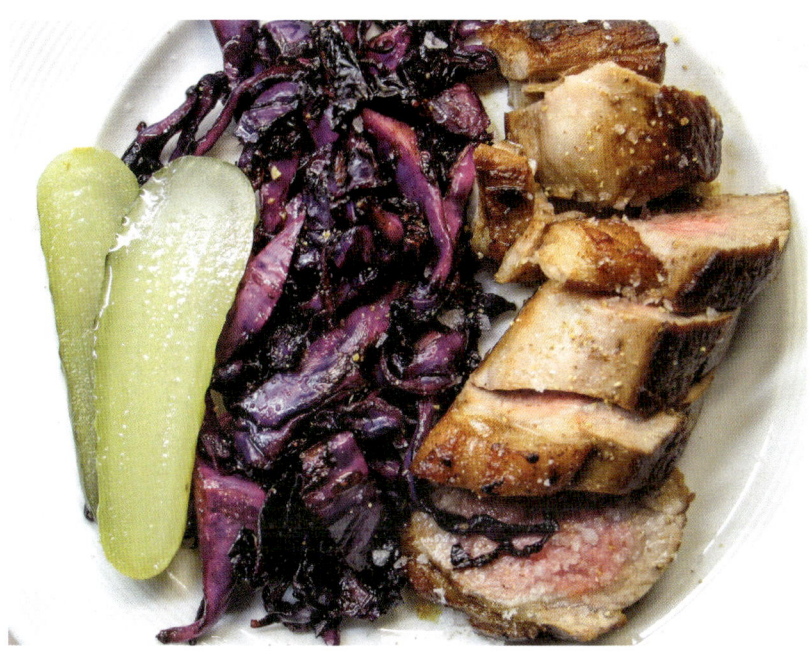

Lamb tenderloin with red cabbage and gherkin

Pan fry the tenderloin whole in olive oil or butter and leave to stand for some minutes, then make inch thick slices.

The red cabbage is fried for 5 minutes in olive oil, with salt, white pepper and a tablespoon of vinegar added halfway.

Pickled gherkins can be hi-carb, so watch out. But you can find low carb versions, and anyway there's less than 10 g of gherkin on this plate which means only about a gram of carbohydrate even with a hi-carb product. As with ketchup, watch the amounts and you'll be fine with the odd hi-carb indulgence.

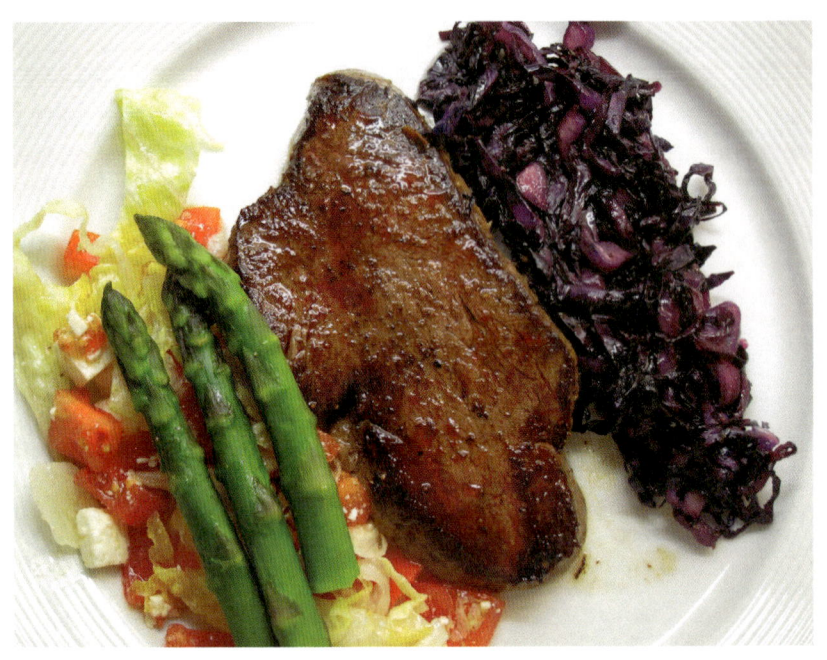

Ribeye steak with red cabbage, asparagus and green salad

The ribeye steak is seared on a hot pan with olive oil for about 2 minutes per side, then left to stand for about 5 minutes.

In those 5 minutes I fry the red cabbage on the same pan, adding a pinch of salt and freshly ground white pepper and a tablespoon of vinegar halfway.

The asparagus are boiled no more than a minute to remain crispy and placed on top of a simple salad of lettuce, tomato and Feta cheese with a simple oil and vinegar dressing.

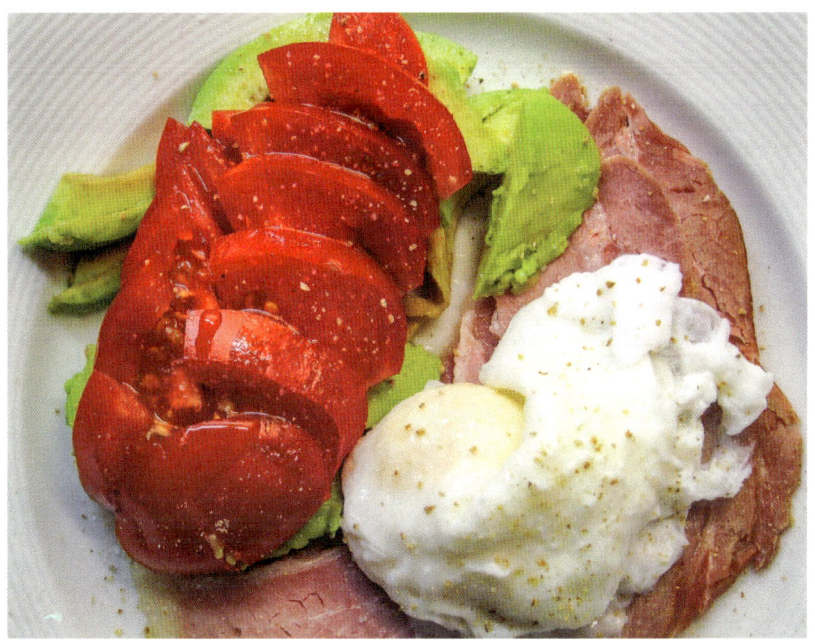

Ham with poached egg, tomato and avocado

Two slices of ham, warmed for 20 seconds in the microwave, with a poached egg on top.

I love eggs but used to only have them poached when eating out. I thought they were difficult to make, but then decided to try and found out that they're not. I break the egg into a cup and gently tip it into vigorously boiling water in not too big a pot, then immediately lower the heat so the water doesn't continue to boil strongly but stays just at boiling point. After 2 minutes 30 seconds I tip it all into a sieve and transfer the egg to the dish.

Before that I've sliced the tomato and half avocado and poured some olive oil over it, maybe my favourite Italian white truffle flavoured kind.

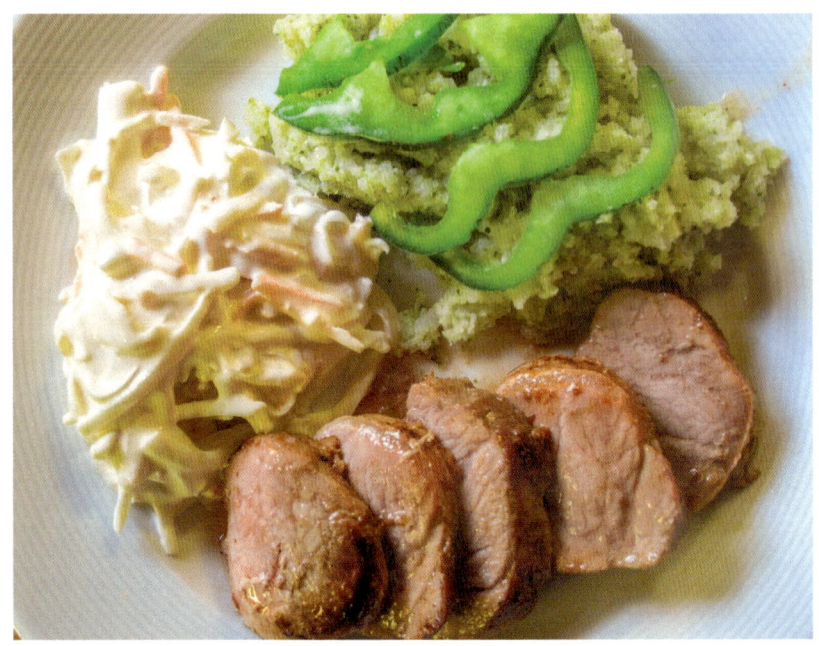

Pork tenderloin with broccoli/cauliflower mash, coleslaw and green pepper

Pan fry the tenderloin whole in olive oil or butter and leave to stand for some minutes before slicing.

The mash is half broccoli, half cauliflower, both boiled quite soft and mashed in a food processor or, if I do large portions, in the large bowl of my Kenwood mixer. I add a knob of butter and maybe a little cream just before serving. This is a tastier and healthier replacement for mashed potatoes.

Top off with green or red pepper and add a dollop of low-carb coleslaw.

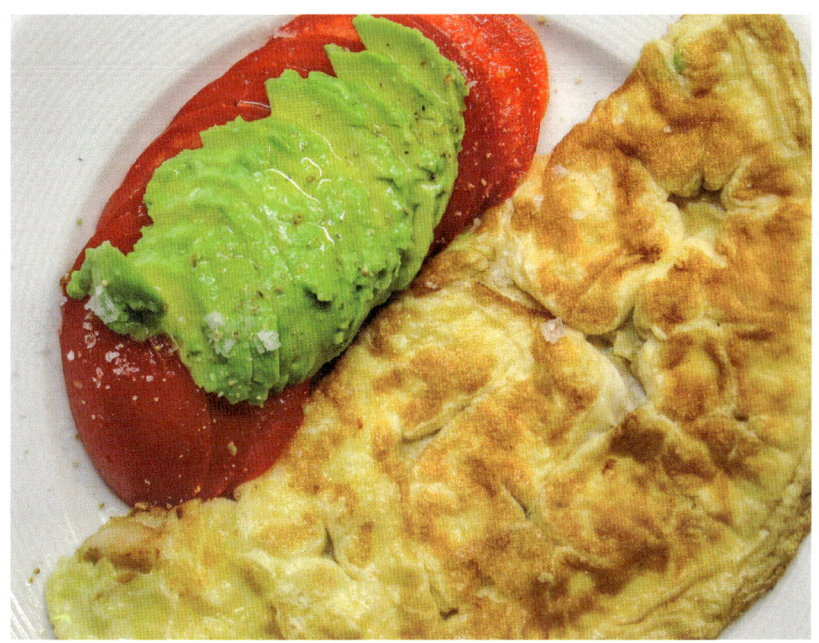

Cheese omelette with tomato and avocado

For once, a two-egg omelette. I gently whisk the eggs with two tablespoons of double cream and two teaspoons of water, then pour them onto a hot pan.

I then add grated cheese, mild or strong as the mood strikes me, over one half of the egg mass, plus a pinch of salt and some freshly ground white pepper. I prefer to close the omelette while it's still quite soft or even runny, but cook it to your own preference.

With that, slices of tomato and half an avocado with salt, pepper and olive oil.

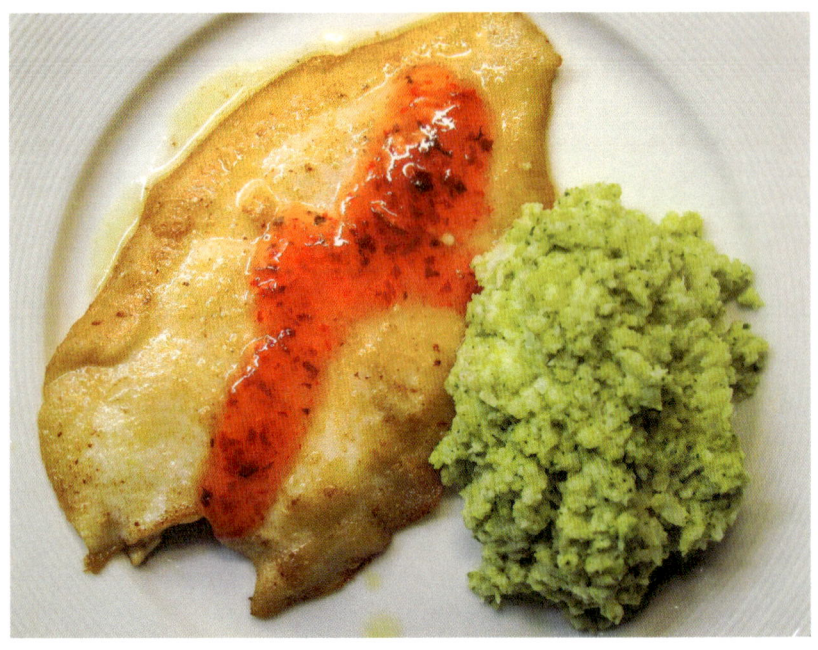

Fried Dover sole with broccoli/cauliflower mash and spicy sauce

The Dover sole is fried gently for about 5 minutes in olive oil, first on the the flesh side, then with the skin side down.

The broccoli/cauliflower mash is my tastier and healthier replacement for mashed potatoes. I often make this in large portions, especially if I have some broccoli that has lost its freshness, and freeze it in portion sized containers for easy re-heating.

The ginger and cayenne sauce is from my fishmonger and almost certainly not low-carb, but hey, there's only a few grams there, so it doesn't make any difference.

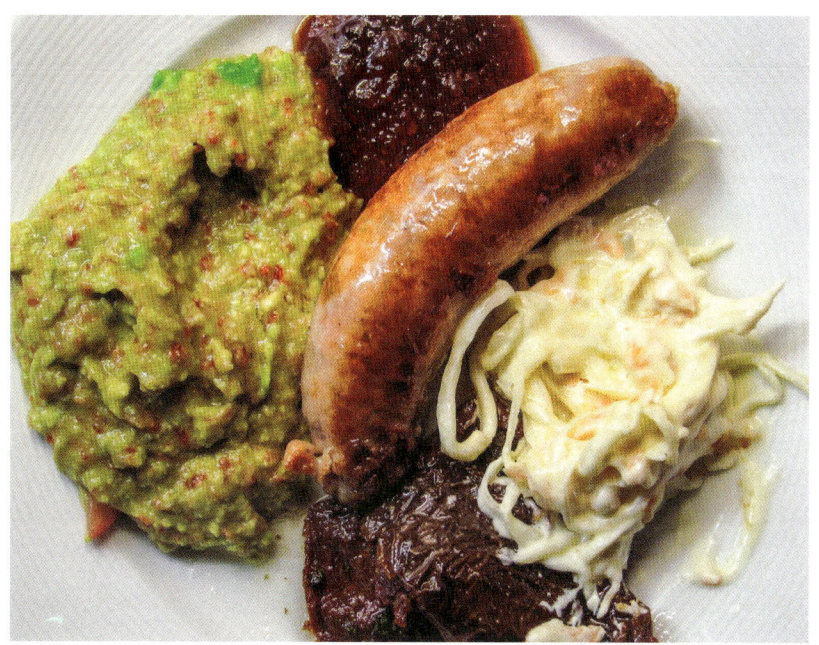

Pork sausage with guacamole, dried tomato, coleslaw and ketchup

Again, this is my own, quick take on guacamole: an avocado, a piece of cucumber and a tomato, all cubed and whizzed for a few seconds in a small food processor with salt, freshly ground white pepper and spices to taste. Use a pinch of cayenne if you want the authentic guacamole bite, but I like mine mild.

The sausage is my local butcher's best low carb, free range pork sausage, and the coleslaw is low-carb from my local deli, as are the dried tomatoes in olive oil.

The ketchup is home made and much lower in carbohydrates than factory ketchup, but as there's just a couple of teaspoons here, it makes little difference one way or the other.

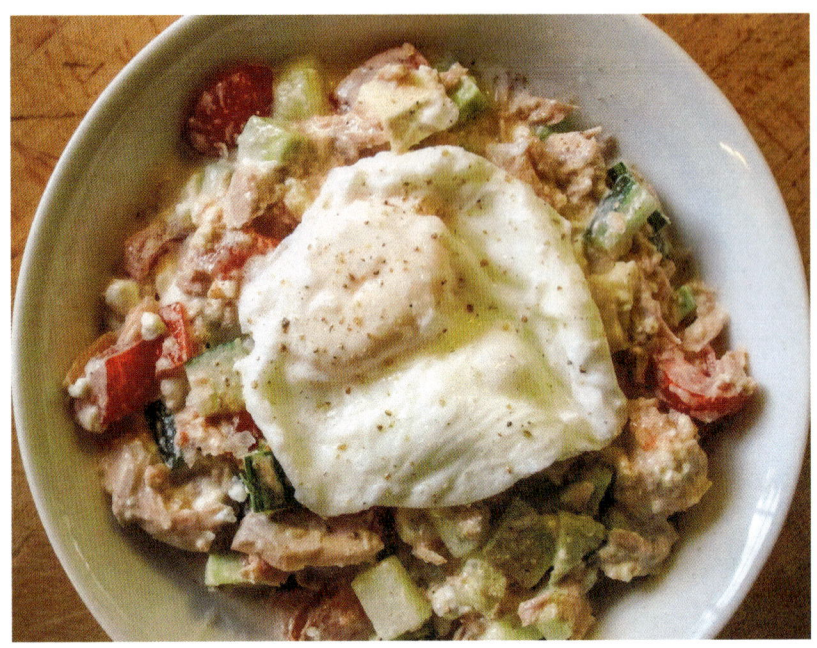

Chicken salad with poached egg

Another no-carb portable lunch. I cube and mix chicken, tomato, cucumber, avocado and Feta cheese with two tablespoons of yoghurt and a tablespoon of creme fraiche, then season with salt and freshly ground white pepper.

Here I have topped it with a poached egg, but use two halves of a hard boiled egg if you make this to go.

Make this fresh in the morning, and it keeps fine until lunch if kept cool. If not, keep the chicken separate and mix it in with the rest just before lunch. The hard boiled egg keeps best in its shell until just before eating, of course.

This no-carb lunch fits neatly into any plastic box with a tight fitting lid, so you can take it with you anywhere.

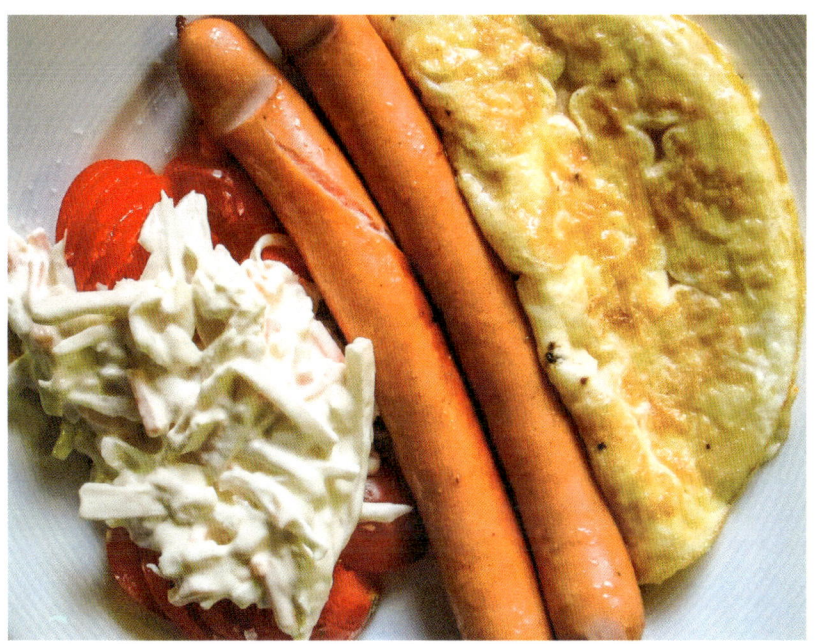

Frankfurters with plain omelette, tomatoes and coleslaw

The frankfurters are quickly fried in olive oil, and the omelette made on the same pan with one egg, a tablespoon cream and a teaspoon water whisked together and seasoned with salt and freshly ground white pepper.

On the side slices of tomato with low-carb coleslaw on top.

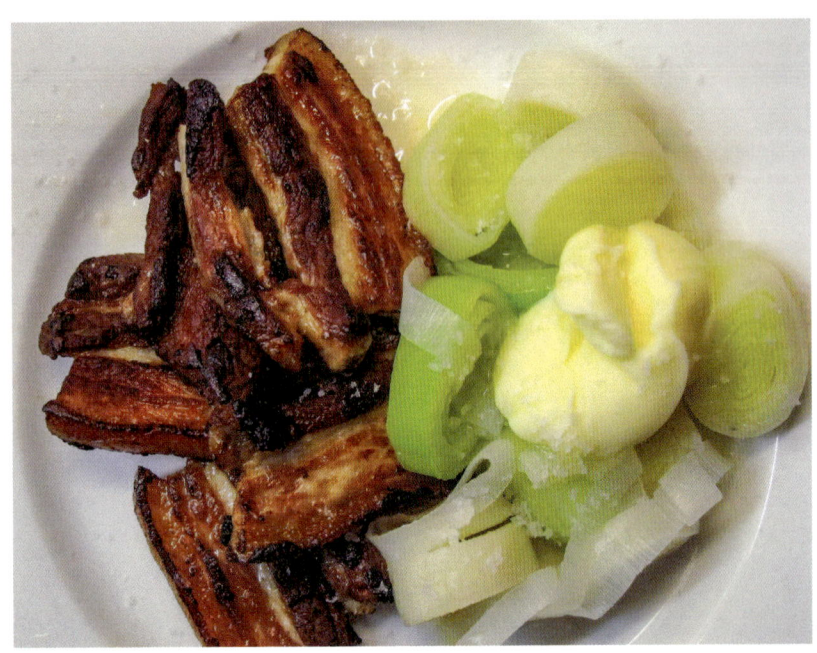

Fried pork belly with boiled leeks and a knob of butter

A no-carb version of a old Nordic dish, traditionally served with potatoes and parsley sauce.

The pork belly is sliced into 6-8mm (¼″) slices and slowly fried on a medium hot pan until crisp. Most of the fat will melt away and what's left should be crisp but tender.

Any vegetables would do but here I chose lightly boiled leeks and just added a knob of butter.

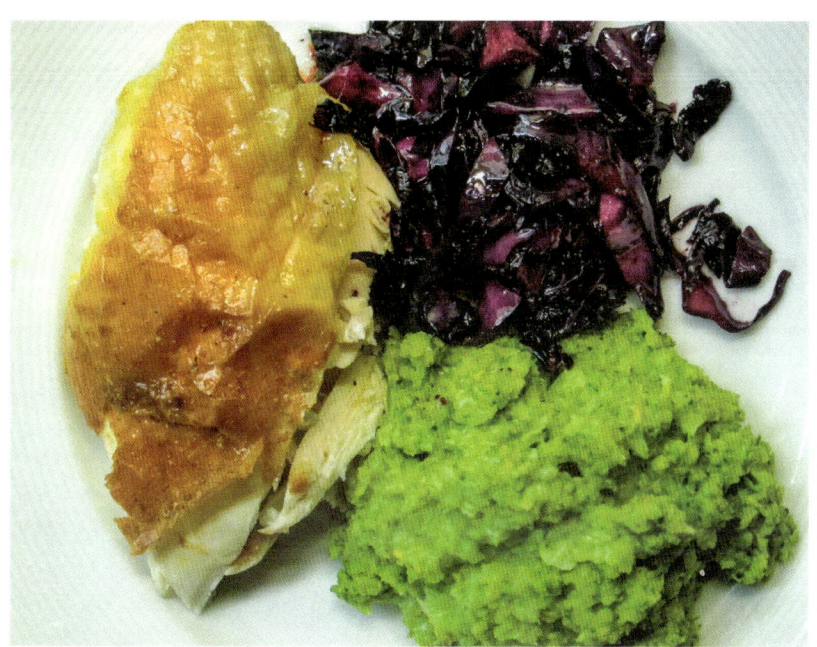

Chicken breast with broccoli mash and red cabbage

I like to roast a whole, free range chicken in the oven and use the various parts for a number of dishes. The breasts go into the "presentation" dishes like here, and lesser cuts can be used in salads or for the simple, childish pleasure of gnawing a drumstick.

My point is that nothing except the bones need go to waste. Even the meat from wings (considered the height of delicacies by some but thrown away my many) and back is delicious in salads.

Here accompanied by my staple veggies: fried red cabbage and broccoli mash.

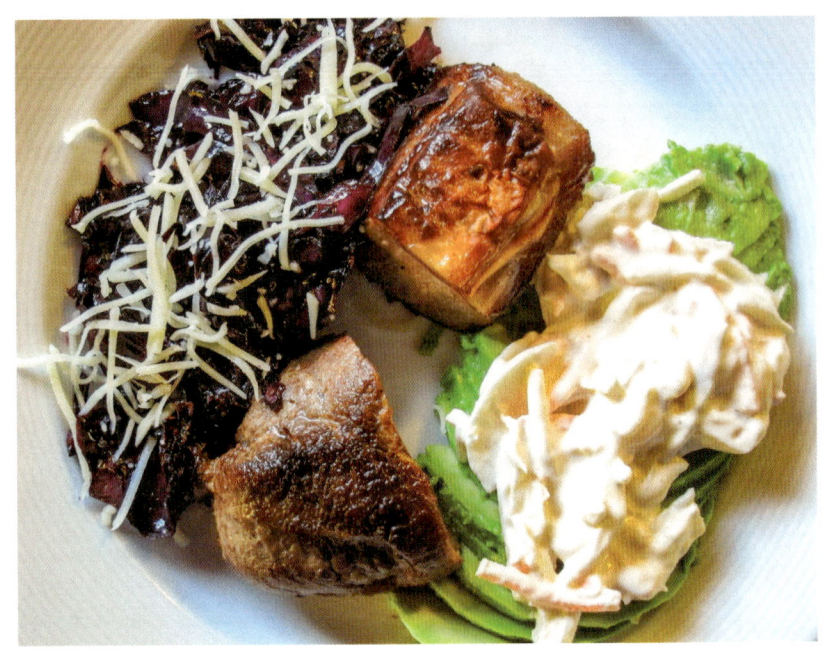

Lamb tenderloin with red cabbage, avocado and coleslaw

This lamb was left over from dinner, so it only needed a little heating on a pan, which I then used to fry the red cabbage in the usual way with only salt, pepper and a little vinegar.

I topped half a sliced avocado with low-carb coleslaw and then got the idea to sprinkle a little grated cheese on top of the cabbage, both for decoration and for taste. It went incredibly well together.

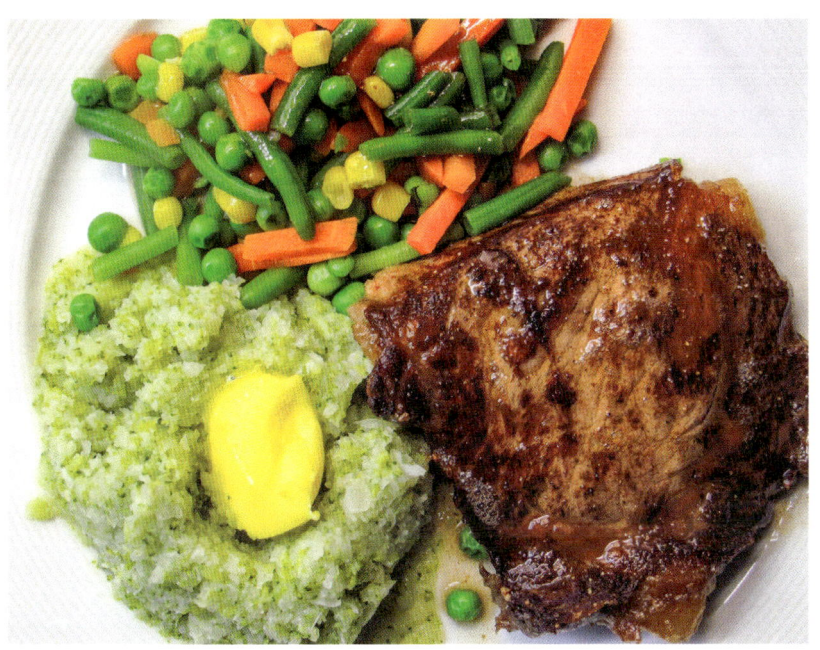

Sirloin steak with broccoli/cauliflower mash and mixed vegetables

I fried this piece of sirloin in a mix of olive oil and butter for about 2 minutes a side, then left to stand.

The mash is my usual broccoli/cauliflower replacement for mashed potatoes, and although peas are a little high in carbs, I do have them occasionally in small amounts.

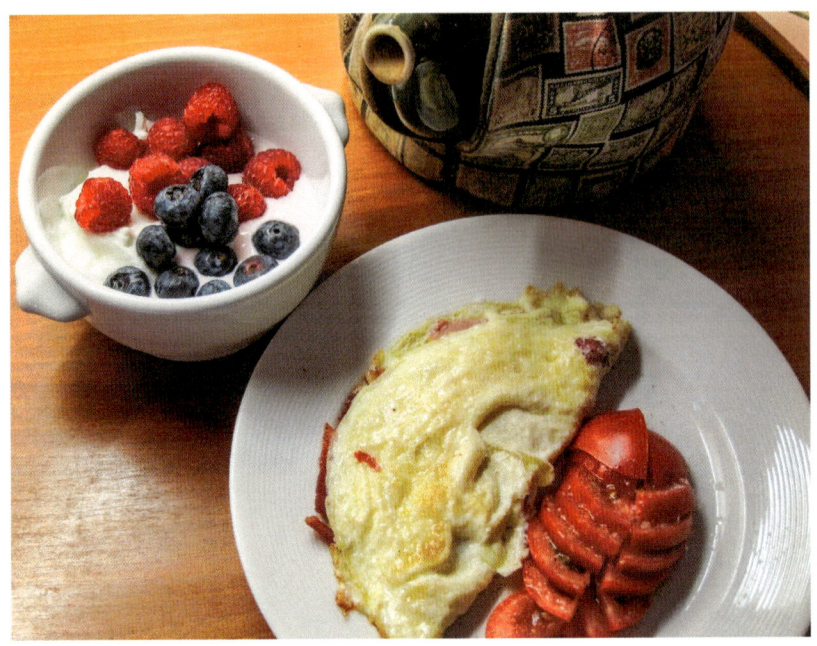

Ham omelette with tomatoes and yogurt with blueberries and raspberries

A treat of a breakfast, so this must have been Sunday. A one-egg omelette full of succulent ham with sliced tomato on the side, and a rare treat of yoghurt with berries.

It's the berries that are naughty here, of course, from a carbohydrate point of view, so the amounts aren't huge but the taste so much more intense for it.

Absolutely no sugar, but I could have added a little cream. The yoghurt is full fat as low fat yoghurt can have twice the carbs as full fat yoghurt. And remember, it's NOT the fat that makes you fat.

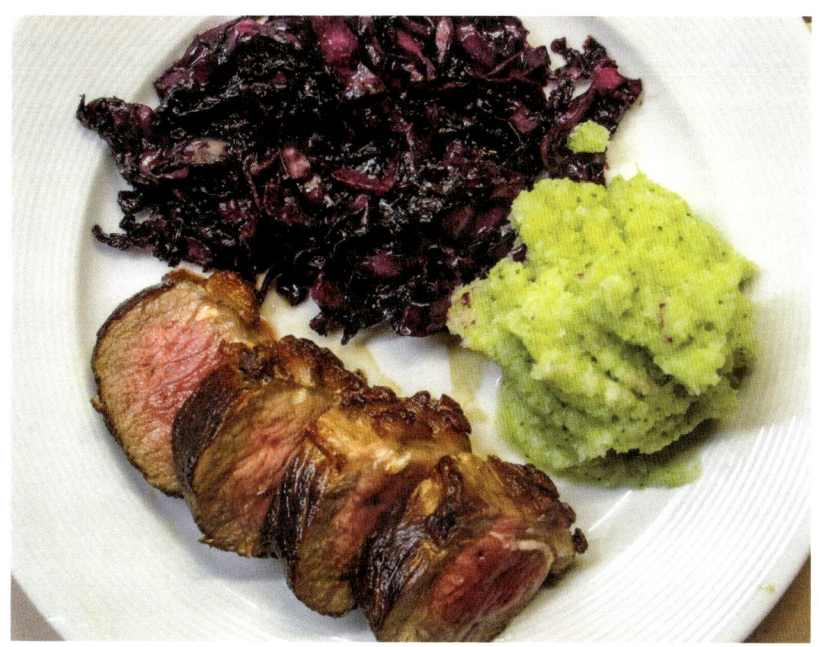

Lamb tenderloin with red cabbage and broccoli mash

Probably the dinner that supplied the leftovers for the lunch three pages ago. Pan fried whole lamb tenderloin with my two favourite, nutritious and delicious vegetables: fried red cabbage and mashed broccoli.

I eat a lot of boiled or steamed, whole broccoli because it's one of the healthiest vegetables in existence with a long list of benefits, from cancer and heart disease to skin protection and detoxification. Look it up.

So the reason you also see a lot of broccoli *mash* in these pictures is that I buy a lot of it, and it sometimes doesn't look its best after a few days, but it's still perfectly good to eat. That's when I mash it and make it look great again.

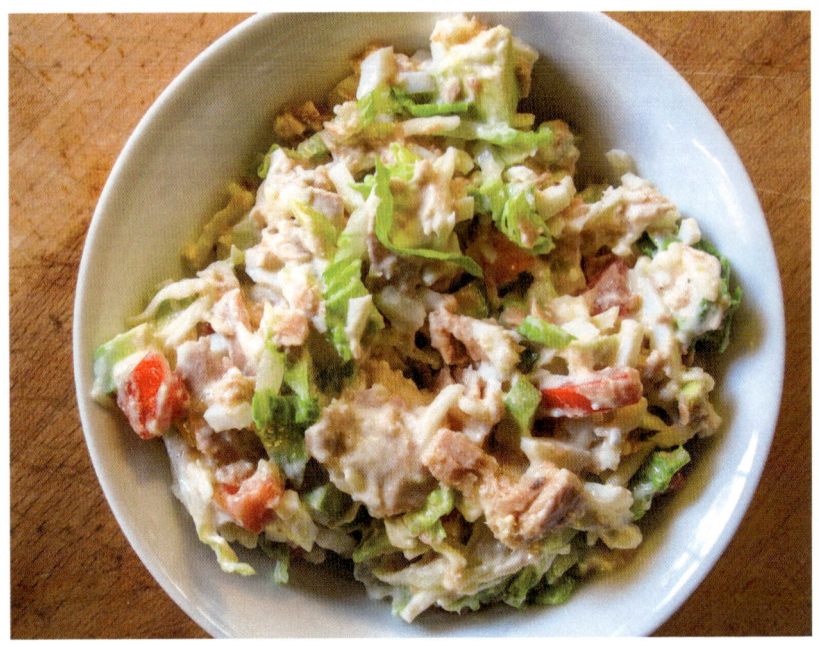

Salmon salad with egg, tomatoes, avocado and lettuce

Like the tuna salad I showed earlier, this salad is made very simply from chopped tomato and avocado, plus in this case salmon of course.

I make a dressing of two tablespoons of yoghurt and a tablespoon of creme fraiche, then mix it and season with salt and white pepper and top it off with lettuce. I could have mixed the lettuce in with the rest, but then it would have been covered in dressing and not look as good. I like my food to look good.

The salmon in this case was the leftovers from last night's dinner, but you can use tinned salmon, and if you are taking this lunch to work and can't refrigerate it that's what you'll want to do in order to keep the fish separate until just before eating.

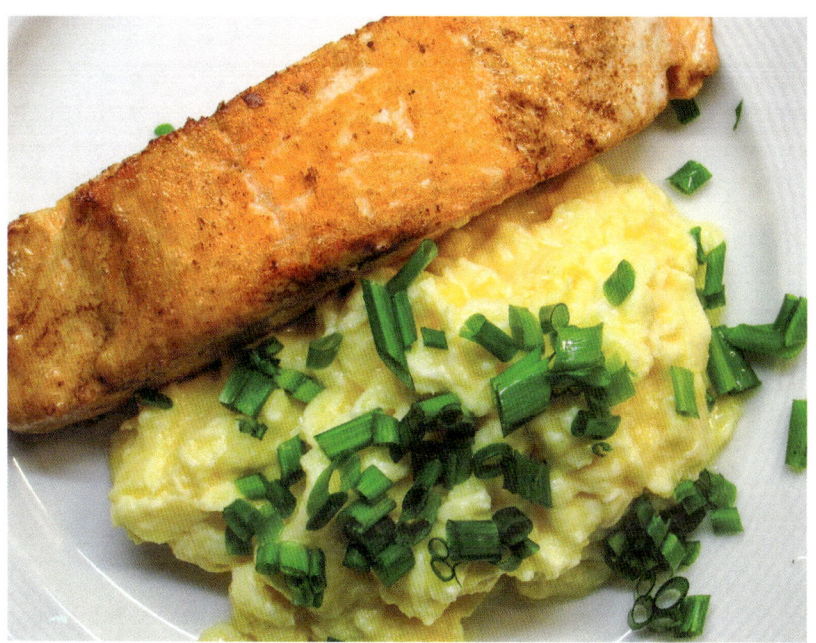

Fried salmon with scrambled eggs and chives

This salmon is fried on a warmer pan than I normally use, in order to create this pretty and crispy surface. After a few minutes I turn down the heat to let the fish cook through.

Served with scrambled egg of two eggs whisked with a little cream and water and topped off with chives.

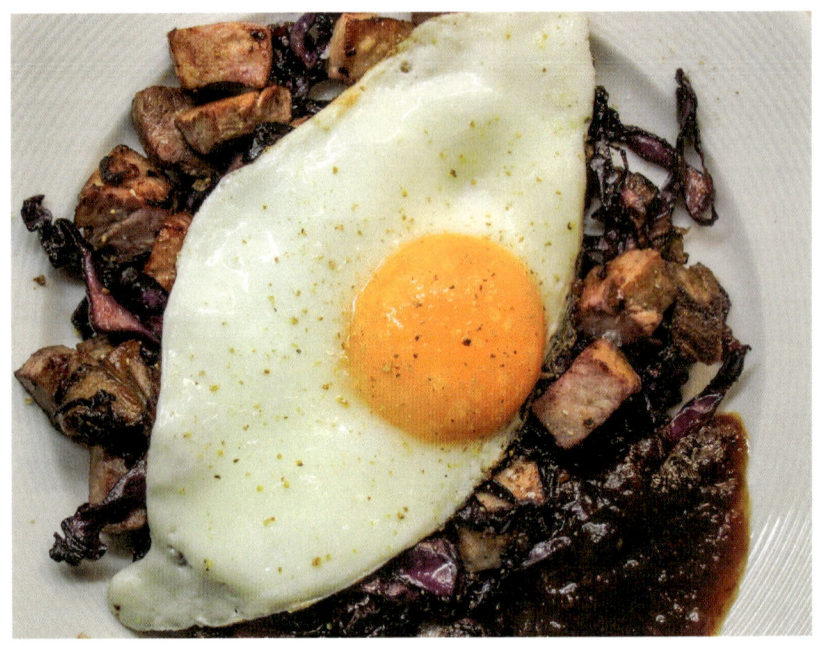

Hash with fried egg and ketchup

This hash, like the earlier one, is made with leftovers, this time beef, and I supplemented with some fresh red cabbage.

Topped off with a fried egg and a couple of teaspoons of home made, relatively low-carb, ketchup on the side.

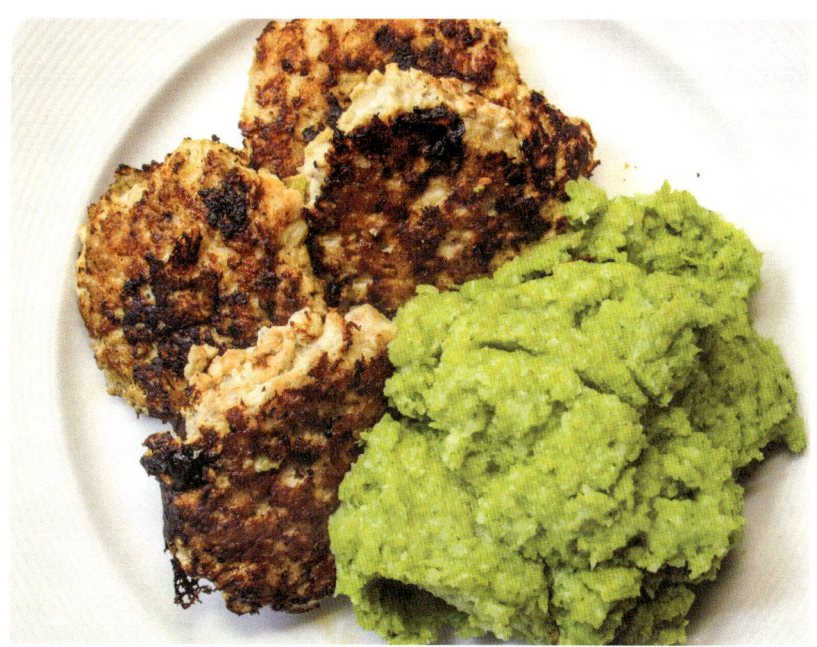

Meatballs with broccoli/cauliflower mash

These are simple, pan fried pork meatballs, but use your own favourite as long as you go easy on the flour or breadcrumbs. I halve the amount of flour in the recipe and use an extra egg to lower the carb content and still keep them together. Beware of processed meatballs as they can contain a lot of flour, so read the label carefully.

A big dollop of broccoli/cauliflower mash balances the fairly rich meatballs nicely. Add a knob of butter if you want.

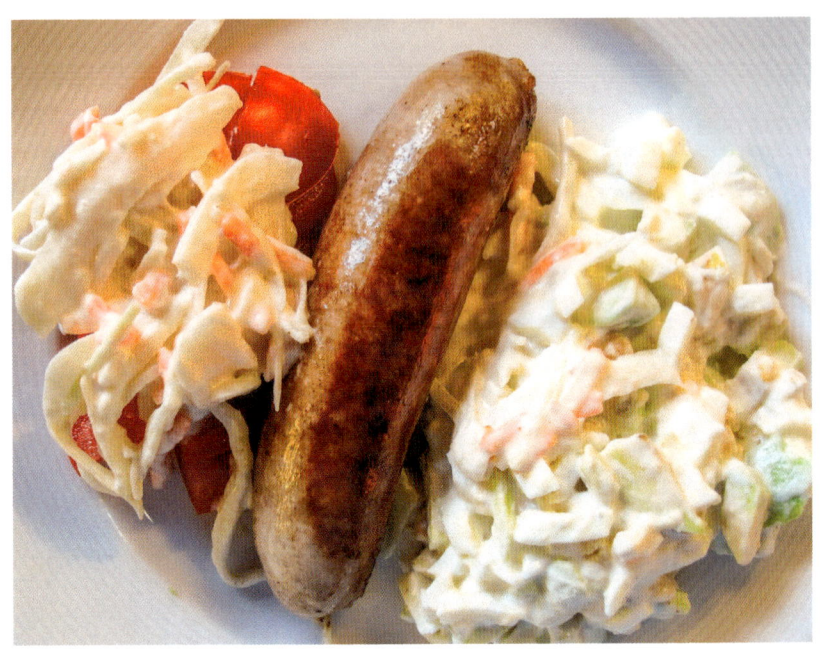

Pork sausage with a salad of egg, avocado and red pepper with tomato and coleslaw

This time my butcher's low-carb pork sausages come with a salad made from a chopped egg, avocado and red pepper with a tablespoon of yoghurt, salt and pepper.

On the other side is my staple diet of tomato and low-carb, full fat coleslaw.

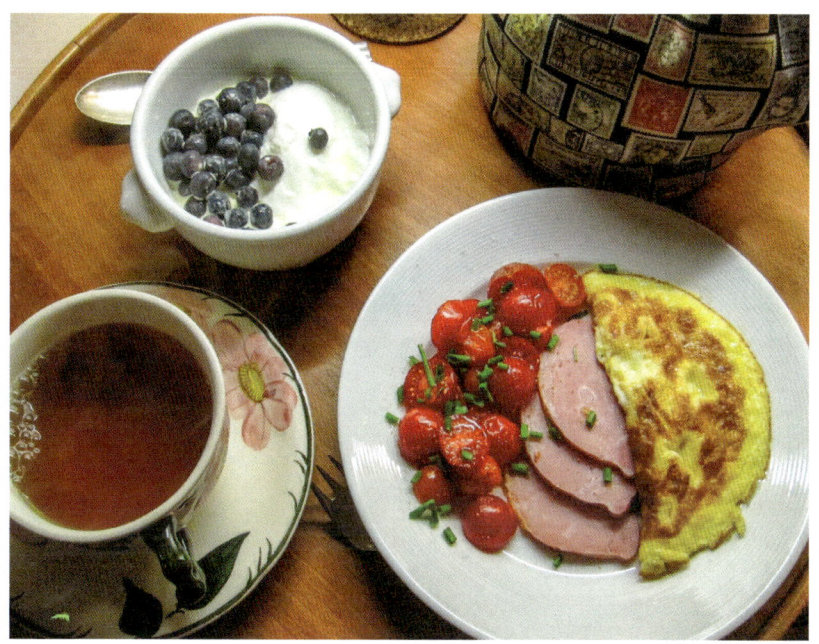

Ham, omelette and tomatoes with yogurt and blueberries on the side

Another indulgence breakfast with slices of succulent ham (in this case home cooked) with a one-egg cheese omelette and tomatoes topped with chives and olive oil.

The indulgence is the yoghurt with blueberries and a little cream on top.

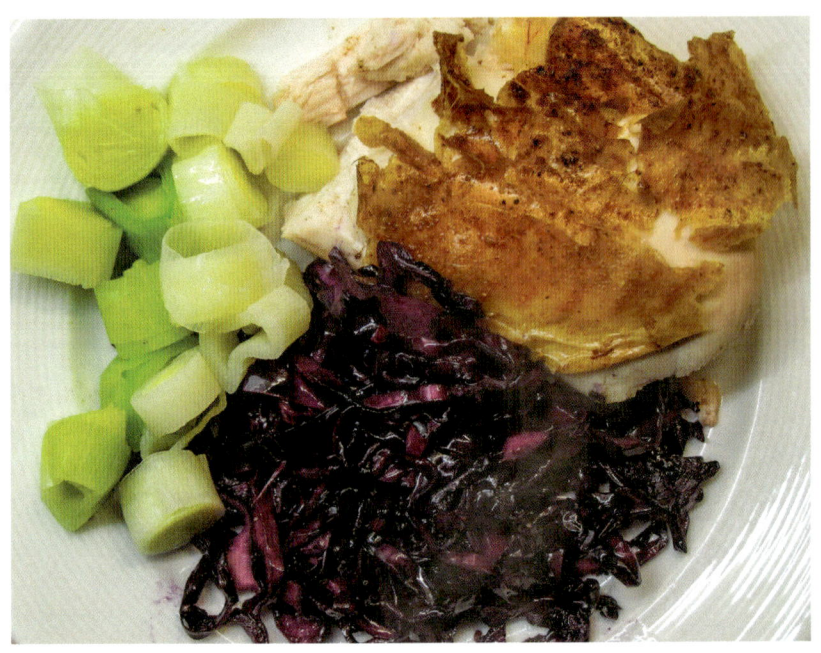

Chicken breast with red cabbage and boiled leeks

The finest cut of an oven fried free range chicken accompanied by pan fried red cabbage and lightly boiled leeks.

As mentioned earlier, I make sure to use every bit of meat from a chicken. That way a more costly free range bird becomes no more expensive than a farmed chicken with a lot going to waste.

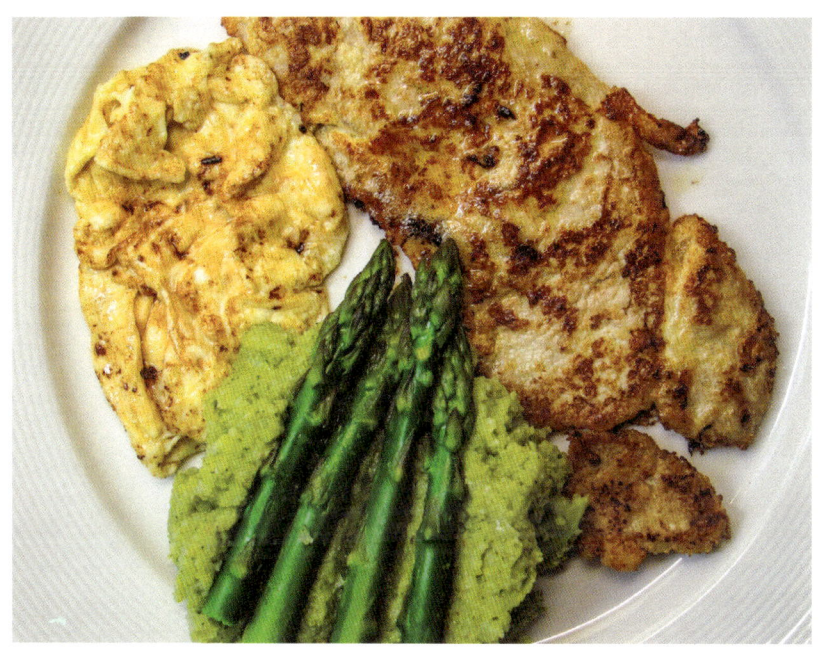

Veal cutlet with asparagus, broccoli mash and scrambled egg

Believe it or not, but this is a no-carb *wienerschnitzel*. Without the breading and without the *bratkartoffeln*, so here is what's left.

I dip the cutlet in an egg whisked with a little cream and water, salt and pepper before frying it, just as I would if I were breading it, I just don't dip it in breadcrumbs afterwards.

With that I serve, in this case, broccoli mash with lightly boiled asparagus on top and the rest of the egg quickly scrambled on the cutlet pan so as not to waste it.

If I had put the traditional anchovy on top (which I haven't in this case), I would have fried it quickly on the same pan to melt it and turn it into more of a sauce.

Admitted, it's not *quite* a wienerschnitzel, but it's delicious in its own right.

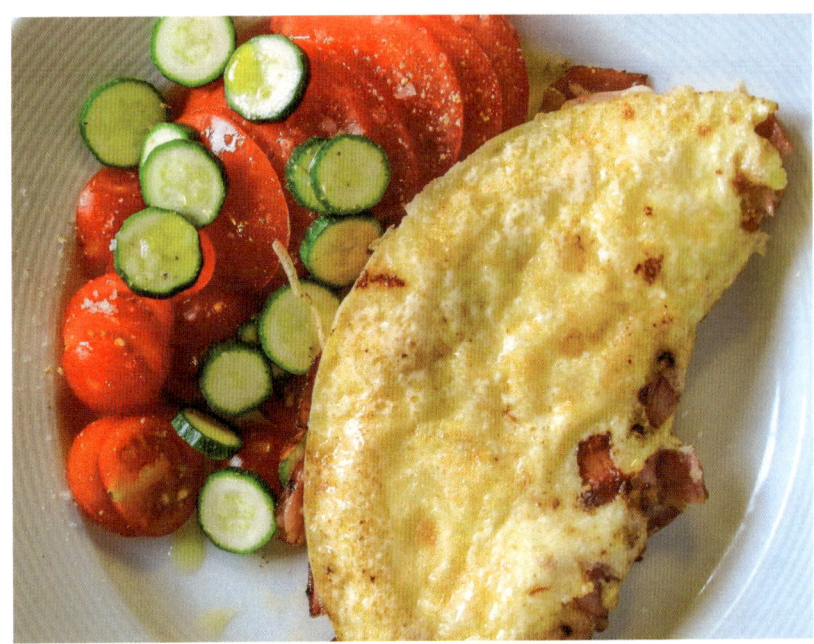

Ham omelette with tomatoes and mini squash

This one-egg omelette full of tender ham with sliced tomato on the side and slices of fresh mini squash is equally appetising for breakfast and lunch.

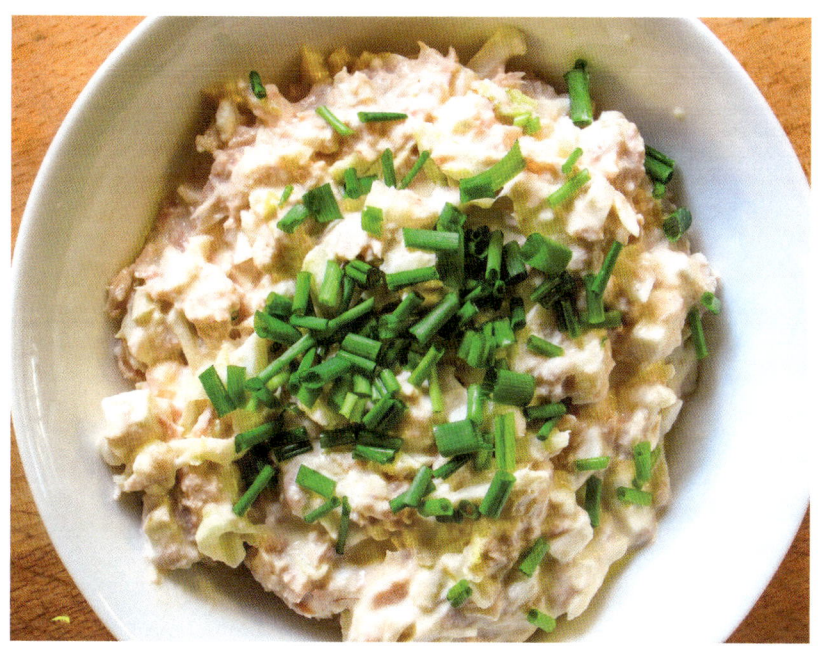

Tuna salad with egg and cauliflower

Another quick and easy to no-carb lunch. A tin of tuna mixed with a chopped egg and cauliflower. The cauliflower can be raw or lightly steamed or boiled as you prefer, but if it is, let it cool completely before mixing.

I make the salad dressing from two tablespoons of yoghurt and a tablespoon of creme fraiche, mixed and seasoned with salt and white pepper and topped off with whatever tasty greenery I have handy.

This is quickly made in the morning, or even the night before, and keeps fine until lunch if you can keep it cool. If not, keep the tuna in the tin and simply mix it in with the rest just before lunch.

Fitting into any plastic box with a tight fitting lid, this lunch is ready to go anywhere you want.

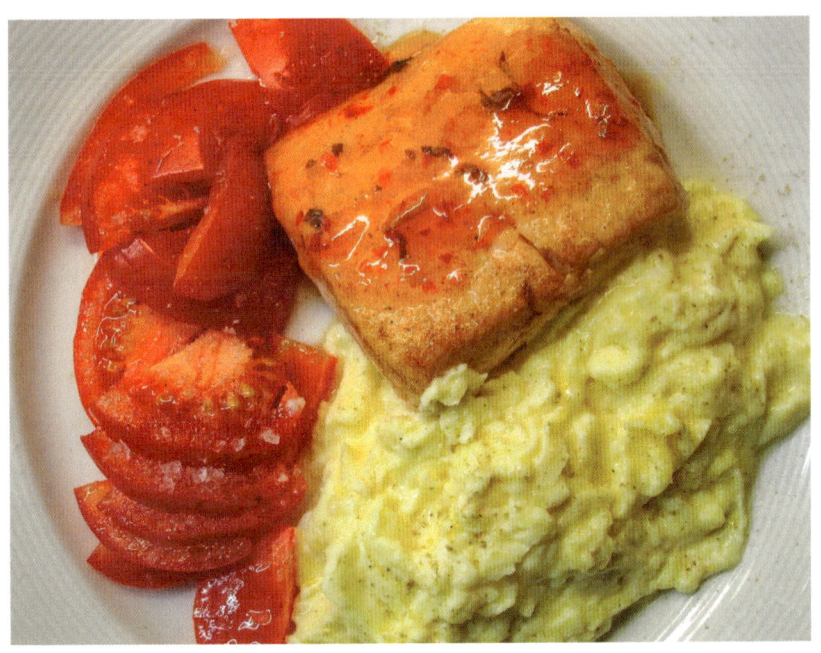

Fried salmon with scrambled eggs and tomato with spicy sauce

Pan fried salmon, again slightly crispy, with tomatoes and scrambled eggs made from two eggs whisked with a little cream and water.

The sauce is the same kind used in earlier menus; not very low carb, but very little of it instead.

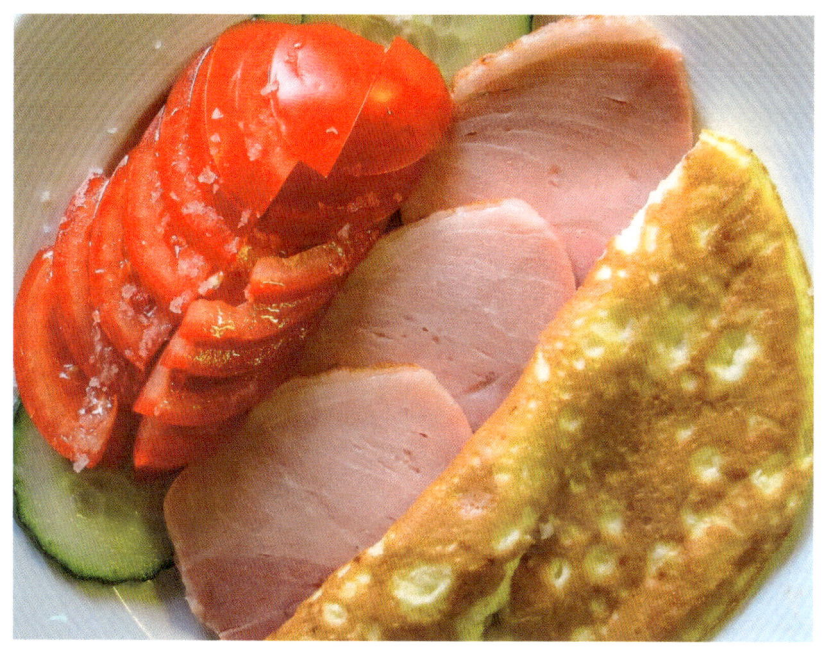

Plain omelette with slices of ham, tomato and cucumber

Slices of home cooked ham with a plain one-egg omelette and a sliced tomato on top of slices of cucumber.

Looks like a lot of the other variations of ham-and-egg that I do, but I do vary both the type of ham and and the accessories, and if I get bored with my food (which, in fact, I don't) all I need to do is take a look at my weight curve.

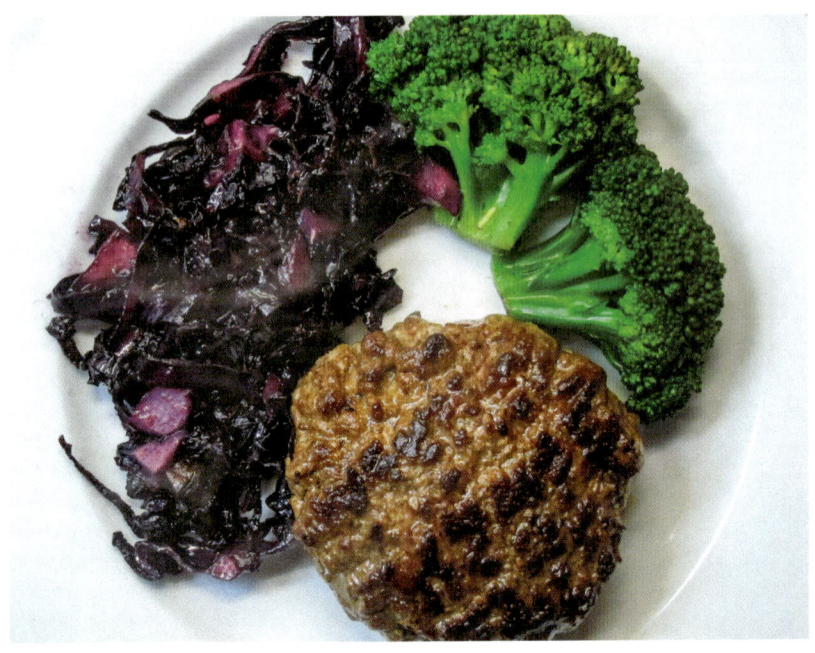

Hamburger with red cabbage and boiled broccoli

This is a home made hamburger with pure, prime minced beef and absolutely nothing else. A world away, health- and taste-wise, from a processed supermarket patty which in some parts of the world contains "pink slime" and goodness knows what else.

I fry it in a mixture of olive oil and butter and serve it with lightly boiled broccoli and my favourite red cabbage, quickly pan fried with a pinch of salt and freshly ground white pepper and a tablespoon of vinegar added halfway.

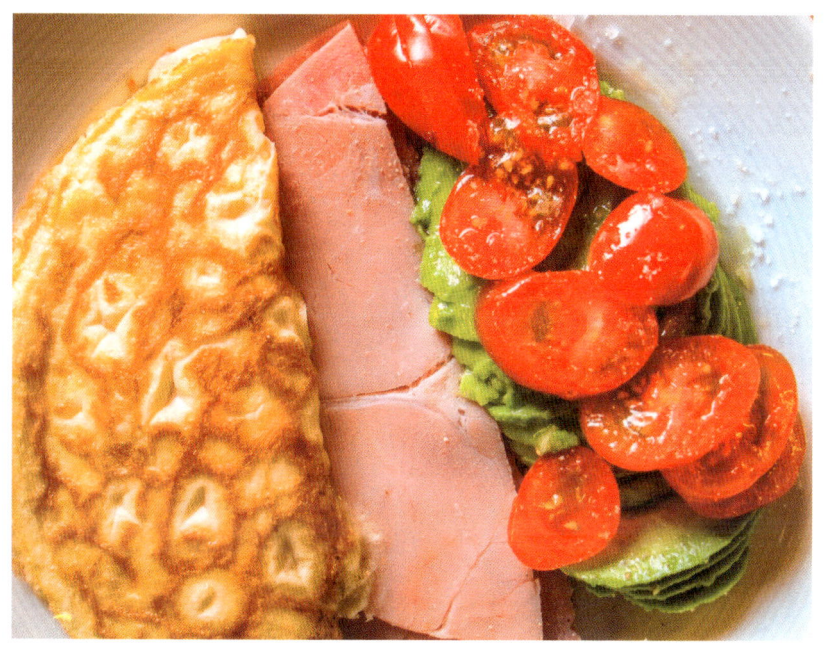

Ham with omelette, tomato and avocado

Slices of ham with a plain, or cheese, one-egg omelette and slices of tomatoes on top of half a sliced avocado.

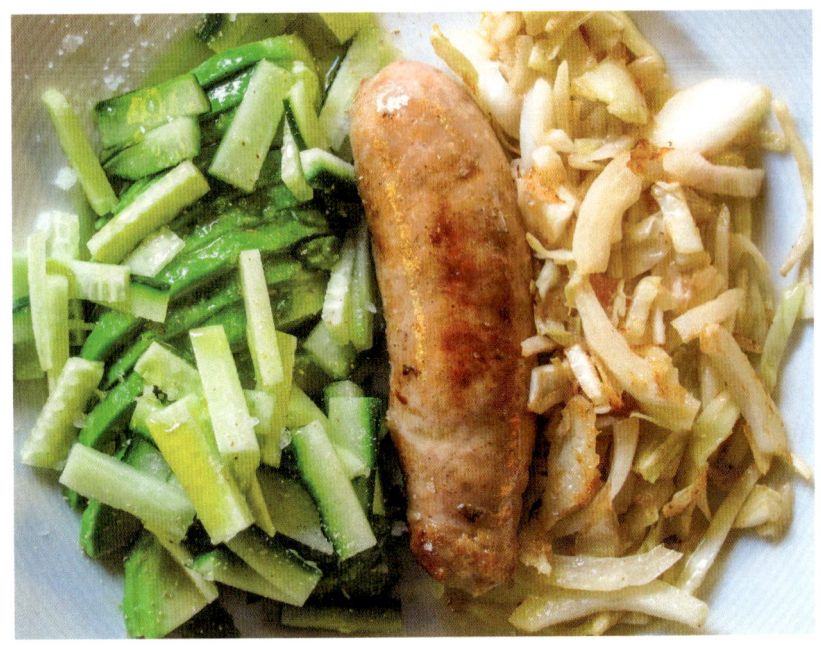

Pork sausage with cabbage, avocado and cucumber

My butcher's best low-carb pork sausage with white cabbage fried with salt, pepper and a tablespoon of vinegar.

On the side half a sliced avocado topped with rods of fresh cucumber.

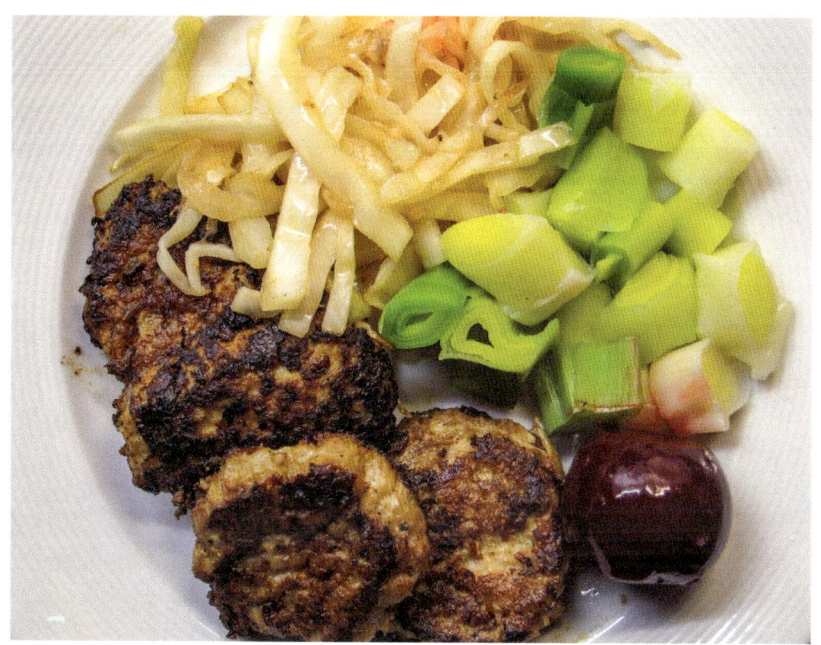

Meatballs with cabbage, leeks and pickled beetroot

I keep my pan fried pork meatballs low carb by halving the amount of flour in the recipe and instead using twice the number of eggs to hold them together. I'm sure you can do something similar to your favourite home made meatballs. Beware of processed meatballs as they can contain a lot of flour, so read the label carefully or avoid them entirely.

The white cabbage is cooked the same way I cook red cabbage: fried 5 minutes in olive oil with salt and freshly ground white pepper, and a tablespoon vinegar added halfway.

In addition lightly boiled leeks and a home pickled beetroot.

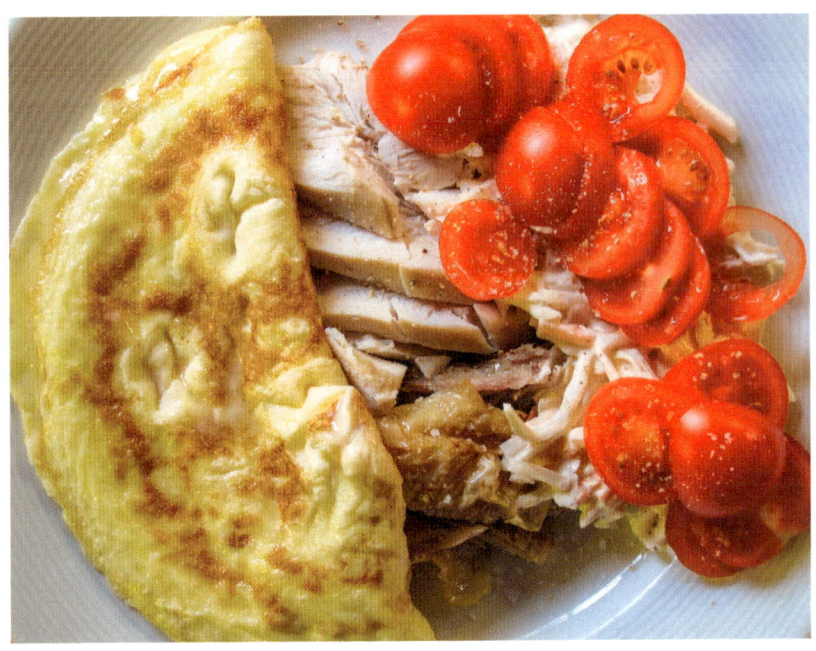

Roast chicken with plain omelette and tomatoes

One of my many chicken dishes, this one is made with slices of chicken breast complemented by a plain one-egg omelette, coleslaw and tomatoes.

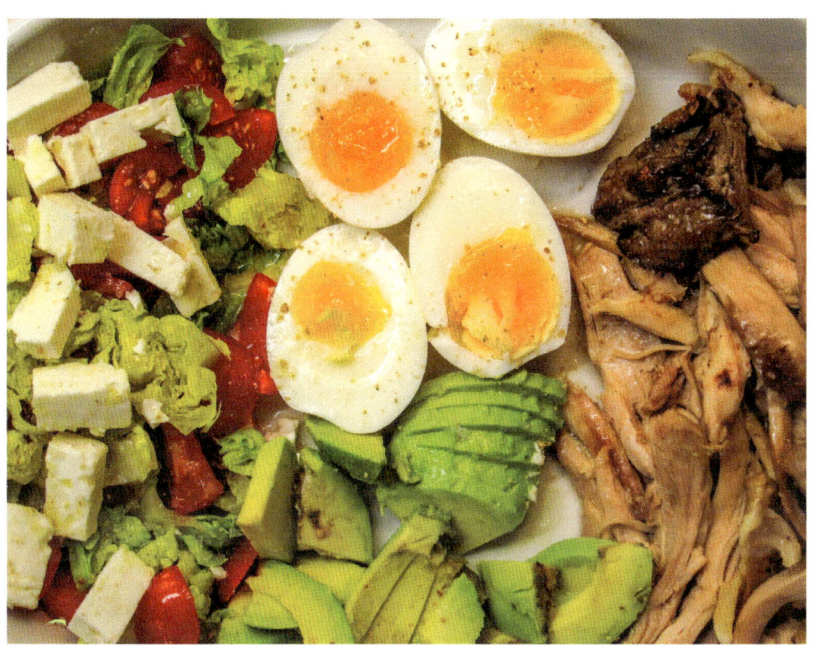

Salad of chicken, eggs, avocado, tomato, lettuce and Feta cheese

When I cook for more than myself, I like to arrange the ingredients of salads separately in a dish so people can compose their own.

Here I serve roast chicken meat with avocado, hard boiled eggs, lettuce, tomatoes and Feta cheese. There's a vinegar-oil dressing on the lettuce, and I have dripped some lemon juice over the avocados. It keeps them from going brown and complements their taste.

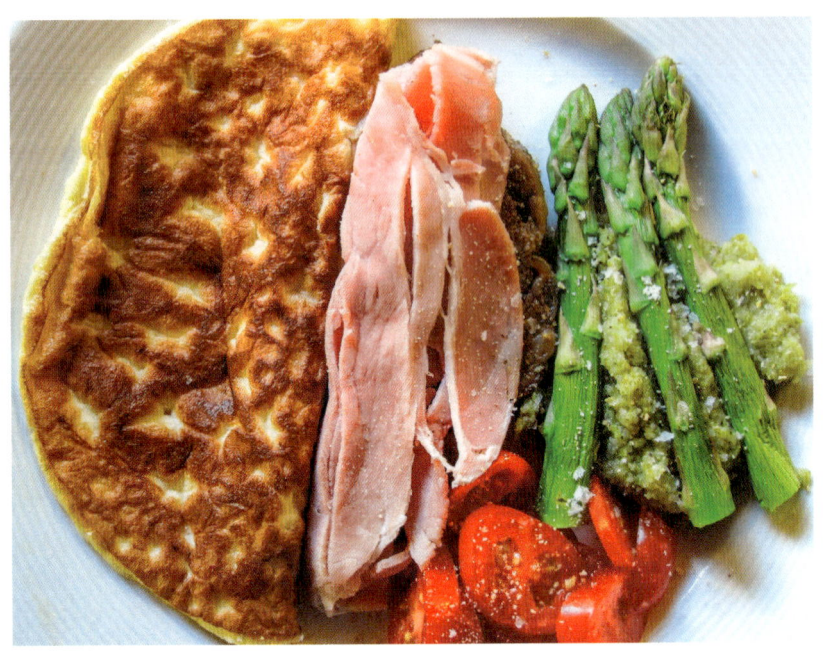

Hamburger with omelette, asparagus, broccoli/cauliflower mash and tomatoes, topped off with ham

Like the previous hamburger, this one is made from prime minced beef, not from a processed supermarket patty. I must have been hungry that day, because I topped it off with a slice of ham.

A plain omelette, lightly boiled asparagus on top of broccoli/cauliflower mash and my beloved tomatoes complete the meal.

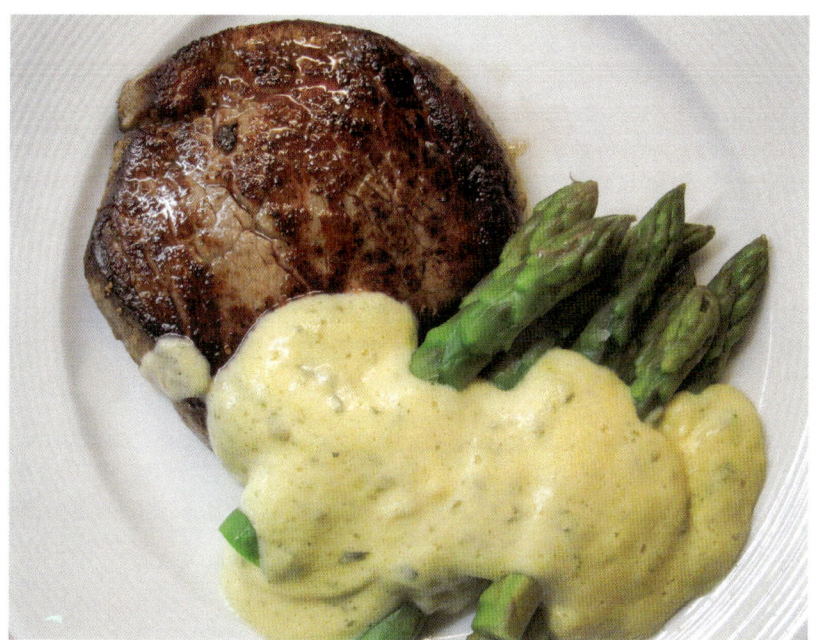

Filet of beef with asparagus and béarnaise sauce

This was for a special occasion: the best local filet of beef, fried in olive oil and butter for 2 minutes a side and served with asparagus boiled al dente and lashings of béarnaise sauce (there was plenty more on the side).

The béarnaise sauce is home made, and I'm tempted to add my recipe here because that's not as simple as everything else in this picture cookbook. But I'm sure you'll have no trouble finding a recipe in your own cookbook or online.

Only please remember that for béarnaise sauce to be the no-carb super delicacy it is, it must be freshly made from nothing but egg yolks, butter, white wine, vinegar, shallots and tarragon, NOT out of a jar or (horror of horrors) made from a mix.

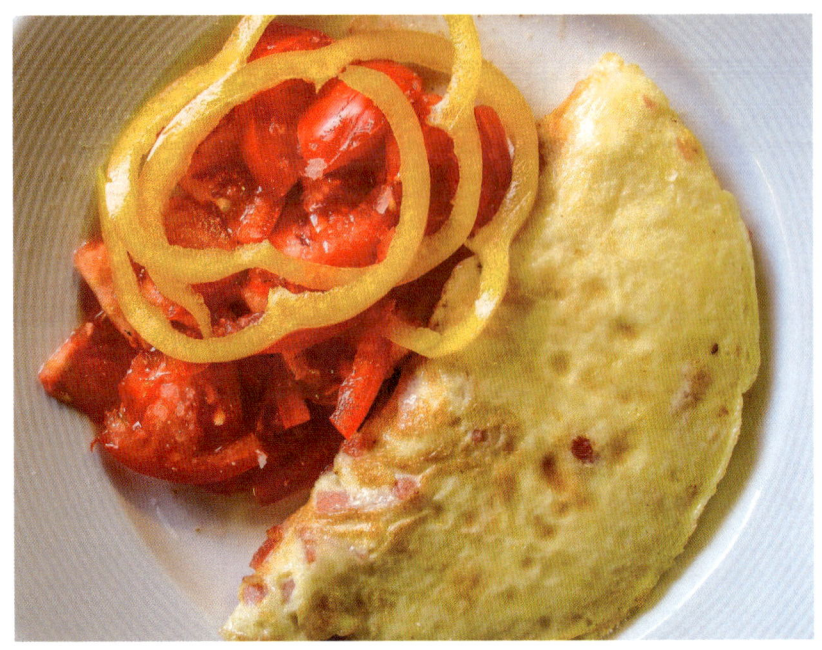

Ham-and-cheese omelette with tomatoes and yellow pepper

A one-egg omelette with shredded ham and cheese with slices of tomatoes and yellow pepper on the side, seasoned to taste with salt and pepper.

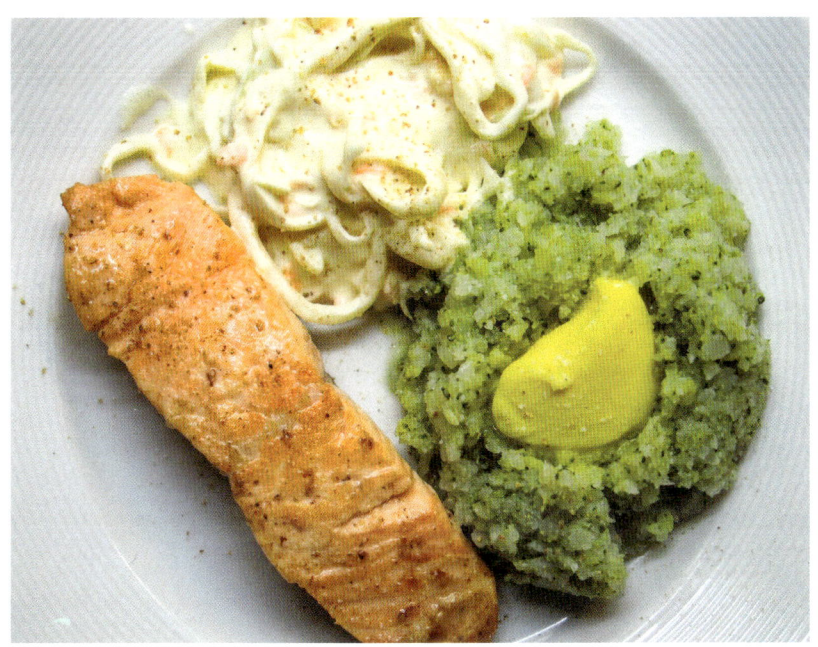

Fried salmon with broccoli/cauliflower mash and coleslaw

This salmon is more lightly fried than in other pictures, by using slightly less heat.

The accompaniment is broccoli/cauliflower mash with a knob of butter and low-carb, full fat coleslaw.

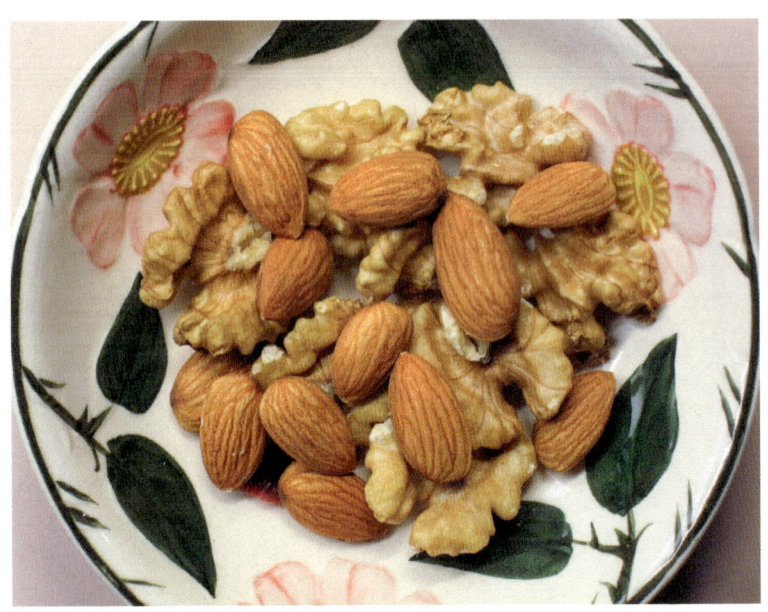

Snack: Walnuts and almonds

This, and sometimes some cheese cubes, are my only occasional between-meals snacks.

Both these nuts are in the yellow band of my carbohydrate list, in other words in a category I'm careful not to overdo, but this amount won't do any harm.

Appendix

I am neither a doctor nor a scientist, or even a journalist trained to research and report on other people's writing, so I have not tried to pretend that I am. Instead, for medical and other background material to what I am saying, I refer you to the following books.

The first of them makes quite a claim in its title: that it can save your life. But as I describe in chapter 2, I have no doubt that it saved mine by making me aware of the link between carbohydrates and health, not just weight.

You would do yourself a favour if you read as many of them as you can get through, and at least the first two. They are all available from Amazon, some for Kindle but at the time of writing others only in print.

Christian B Allan & Wolfgang Lutz:

Life Without Bread

How a Low-Carbohydrate Diet Can Save Your Life

ISBN 978-0658001703

Barry Groves:

Trick and Treat

How Healthy Eating is Making Us Ill

ISBN 978-1905140220

Dr Malcolm Kendrick:

The Great Cholesterol Con

ISBN 978-1844546107

Uffe Ravnskov:

Fat and Cholesterol are Good for You

ISBN 978-9197555388

Hannah Sutter:

Big Fat Lies

Is Your Government Making You Fat?

ISBN 978-1906821371

Blood glucose and ketone metering

Many different glucose meters are available, both online and at your local chemist, so you don't need my help to find one.

Ketone meters are a little harder to find, so I am including details of the meter I am using, which measures both glucose and ketones in the blood (using two different kinds of test strip).

Test strips for measuring ketones in urine are easy to find, but less accurate than measuring it in the blood because they rely on the amount of ketones being excreted, and that varies for a number of reasons.

FreeStyle Optium Neo Blood Glucose and Ketone Monitoring System from Abbott Diabetes Care, 666 Doncaster Road, Doncaster VIC 3108, Australia, www.abbottdiabetescare.com.

You are unlikely to find this in your local shops (unless you happen to live in Doncaster, Victoria), but both the meter and the strips are available in several popular online shops.

No, I don't get a commission, I just like their system, and it's the only one I know of that does both glucose and ketones.

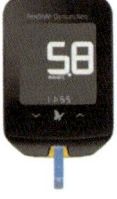

Made in the USA
Charleston, SC
11 March 2015